FAITH, FRIENDSHIP, & FERTILITY

Navigating the Journey to Motherhood

Tenisha Patterson Brown
DeShaun Wise Porter
Rayan Marks

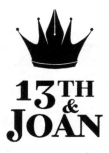

13TH & JOAN

For permission requests, write to the publisher, addressed "Attention: Permissions Coordinator," 205 N. Michigan Avenue, Suite #810, Chicago, IL 60601. 13th & Joan books may be purchased for educational, business or sales promotional use. For information, please email the Sales Department at sales@13thandjoan.com.

Printed in the U. S. A.

First Printing, September 2023.

Library of Congress Cataloging-in-Publication Data has been applied for.

ISBN: 978-1-953156-40-2

We dedicate this to every person suffering in their journey
and most importantly to:

Our grandmothers, who covered us with prayer since birth
and encouraged us to never quit;

Our children. You are our ancestors' wildest dreams.
Everything we do is for you; and

Our angel babies.
We will forever hold you close.
We love you.

ACKNOWLEDGEMENTS

To our husbands, who remained resolute in faith, held our hands, dried our tears, and showed us unconditional love through every success and every challenge on this journey. We love you, and we thank you.

To our parents, who prayed relentlessly for our prayers to be answered and for our health to prevail. It is our greatest honor to continue to make you proud. Thank you for raising us to be the women we are and are still becoming.

To our sister friends, who supported us, encouraged us, and loved us even when our physical presence may have wavered in this process.

To our infertility family members, whether you're researching your options, currently on the in vitro fertilization (IVF) journey, have had success or know someone going through the process—thank you. We have drawn hope, strength, and inspiration from each of you in different ways. We hope our transparency blesses someone else.

Tenisha Patterson Brown, Esq.,
DeShaun Wise Porter,
and Rayan Marks

"We delight in the beauty of the butterfly, but rarely admit the changes it has gone through to achieve that beauty."

– Dr. Maya Angelou

CONTENTS

PREFACE

This book is a compilation of our stories over a period of six years. Between the start of new business ventures, promotions, relocations, monumental losses (grandmothers and children), milestone birthdays, doctors' appointments, IVF protocols, and life in general, we each had moments where the words flowed like a river and other times when the tears would soak the keyboard but not a word was written. We have collectively fought through those tears in an effort to not abandon telling our story.

The journey to parenthood through fertility treatments is not a path less traveled, however, it is less discussed. Through our transparency, struggles, and triumphs, we hope that someone can draw hope. In moments of despair, we are striving to deliver strength. And in the beautiful moments of success, we hope to inspire others to tell their story to ignite a flame in someone to try again, if that is what it takes. Most importantly, we want this to serve as a reminder that no one is alone on this journey.

HER Story

"Blessed is she who believed, for there
shall be a fulfillment of those things
which were told her from the Lord."
- Luke 1: 45 NKJV

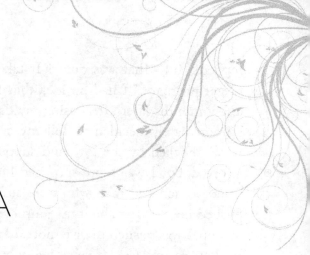

TENISHA

"...Be strong and courageous. Do not be afraid;
do not be discouraged, for the Lord your
God will be with you wherever you go."
– Joshua 1:9 NIV

My story was unexpected to say the least. At 29, I had no idea that I would face the toughest battle of my life. From day one, I was moved to transcribe my journey and, most importantly, my feelings. It is important to tell my story because I believe that my purpose is to connect and support women who have suffered a loss or are struggling with infertility. When I started my journey to motherhood, I had no idea what to expect. I was bright-eyed and bushy-tailed. I was blessed to get pregnant after my first cycle of IVF and I was overjoyed, but honestly, I was shocked that at 29 I had to even resort to IVF to conceive. As I walked out of my last appointment before being transferred to my regular OB/GYN, the front desk receptionist asked me when I was coming back, and I told her that I was pregnant. She replied with "That was quick! It takes other women years to get pregnant." I had no idea that I would see her again a few months later after losing my daughter. After the loss, I immediately decided to tell my story through my blog. I was shocked by the love and support my husband and I received, but I was more surprised by the private messages from women and men who were suffering in silence. God pushed me to write about my journey and every time I tried to stop, I was pushed to give more. I know that it is a part of my journey, and God is using me to help other women. I feel like God put it on my heart to share.

Too often women suffer in silence due to the stigma associated with being "infertile." There is a sense of guilt and a sense of failure. There is also the stigma about being less than a woman because you can't or haven't been able to have children. It's frustrating and hurtful all at the same time. I never accepted the guilt, but unfortunately most women do. Most women who have suffered a pregnancy loss or struggled to get pregnant have encountered those frustrations. The goal of this narrative is to help people understand that we—women who struggle with fertility--don't want pity, we just want people to be mindful of what some women go through. Quite frankly, it is never appropriate to ask a woman why she doesn't have kids. The physical aspect of infertility is difficult, but the most taxing part for me was having to explain repeatedly to those I love what I am going through. My goal each time I share my journey is to help eliminate the feeling of being alone for others enduring similar journeys. Too many women suffer in silence. Too many women feel like this is a battle they face alone. It's not embarrassing and unfortunately, it has become a very common issue with younger women. The most difficult factor about telling my story is getting unsolicited advice about how I should get pregnant and stay pregnant. Most of them are judgmental comments that are based on ignorance about my story. The most rewarding factor about telling my story is counseling other women through their faith walk while they are moms-in-waiting.

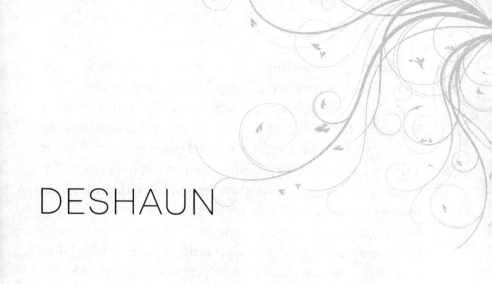

DESHAUN

"Therefore, I tell you, whatever you
ask for in prayer, believe that you have
received it, and it will be yours."
– Mark 11:24 NIV

FOR YOU AND ME

If I had a penny for the times I've heard *"Time heals all wounds,"*
I'd be rich. Not filthy rich, but certainly a step beyond comfortable. Time helps, I agree, but additional work is needed
to truly heal. For me, telling my story is a way to heal myself
while helping others. The journey to motherhood is a unique
one for all women, but when met with challenges in con-
ceiving, the journey can be a lonely one. It can be difficult
knowing where to turn, what to say, how to act, and some
days, how to put one foot in front of the other to keep going.
It is my hope that my story will provide both comfort and
hope to someone else on a similar journey.

Many may say sharing my story is courageous, but I'd argue there is both beauty and courage in the actual writing of the story. Surviving miscarriages and failed IVF transfers while managing the whims of daily life is painful and exhausting on its own, but I personally struggled to write many chapters because I felt like I was reliving the pain all over again. *Is it cathartic?* Yes, one can say that. *Painful?* Yes, that too. Both feelings can co-exist. There are so many women I know who have endured this journey in complete silence, and if it wasn't for my very courageous friend, Tenisha, I too may have fallen into that category. As a private person, my long*er* road to motherhood is one that is being lived out on a public stage, unintentionally. Unintentional because when you check certain boxes in life, it becomes very hard to completely avoid certain questions. For me, I checked the box of having been married for three years *and* over the age of 35, so hence, the question about kids was usually unavoidable. Sometimes it was a straight to the point, TKO-type questions, and other times it was delivered in a circumspect way, but either way unavoidable. Either way, intrusive. Either way, hurtful and for me, unintentional. Family and close friends knew of our desires so in the absence of a baby bump or cooing baby boy or girl, it became easy to anticipate the question, heartbreaking to answer it, but completely impossible to avoid it. Thus, I had to own it. I surely didn't pick this battle. If life was a series of multiple-choice options, I definitely wouldn't have picked it, but here I was. Here we were, and if I couldn't avoid it, I had to find the *silver tint* and for me, that was telling my story with hopes that it will help someone else not feel alone. Not feel inadequate. Not feel hopeless.

Let me not oversell it. I still chose my moments to tell my story. LikeI said, this book took years to create. I was not courageous *everyday*. It took me months to deal with the pain of my first miscarriage. It was then that I realized just how many women suffer the loss of their baby(ies) in silence. Suffer through the IVF journey in silence. Silence because it's hard to talk about. Silence because talking makes it real and the real hurts. Silence because words do no justice to the pain. Silence because *you* wouldn't understand. Silence because the disingenuous positivity with no facts is old. Silence because the statistics told me this shouldn't be a problem. Silence because who wants to be the Debby-downer. Silence because since childhood you may have been taught to "brush yourself off and keep going." Silence. Because. For whatever brings the silence, it is there, and it is real. And the *real* hurts. Bad. Knowing and hearing the stories of other women on a similar journey can take that silence to a whisper and then to a conversational level where we can breathe faith and courage into and over one another.

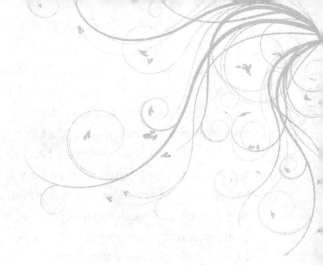

RAYAN

"With God first, you will not fail!"
– Unknown

M Y HOPE IS THAT SOMEONE HEARING MY STORY CAN actually be prosperous. Going through this experience, I wish someone would have told me that having a baby is not that easy. Becoming a mother is really a blessing, and it is not as easy as it seems.

I grew up in a small town and when people get pregnant, it is looked upon as a negative versus a blessing. That is what I have always known until I grew up and moved on. To me, a child is a miracle because not everyone is blessed to have children. Through the process of writing this book, I have learned that of course, there are more women than I have known who are experiencing this issue. Infertility used to be a discussion that was not spoken on but now that we are writing this book, I am starting to see more women coming forth with their story and their journey. It seems like every time I pick up a book or when I look at social media, that is what's on my timeline.

There are so many women going through the same journey in silence. Women like me, who go through this, want to feel their baby move for the first time. It's something we anticipate but unfortunately, struggle to experience. Many women suffer in silence because it's so hard to face the pain and not feel like a failure. When women have devastating moments, I believe we go into a state of depression and seek ways to comfort ourselves. I dealt with my devastation with food. I went from weighing 145 pounds to 175 pounds in less than a year. IT was difficult. Now that I can, I want to tell my story, and I believe that the many women struggling on their journeys to motherhood will be the most impacted by my story. There are so many going through the same trials and living in silence.

I believe this chance is really God-sent because hearing another woman's story would remind me and let me know I am not alone. I hope my testimonies and stories can help at least one woman faithfully, spiritually, and inspirationally on this journey to motherhood. It took me months to write my stories because my heart would endure the pain every time I planned to complete my stories. As I wrote, I cried, I laughed, and just tried to enjoy the good moments. That's really how you have to go through the process. Reading other women's stories and talking about my experience has been very therapeutic and kept me sane. It's ok to be frustrated, feel defeated in the moment, angry, disappointed, and drained. We all go through our hard times. But at the end of the day, we still must keep the faith that we will be future mothers. God is not saying no, He is just saying not right now. The most difficult factor about telling my story is reliving the pain and missing my angels even more, but the most rewarding factor is being able to write about it. It has helped me tremendously.

The
Walk of Faith

"For with God nothing
will be impossible."
—Luke 1:37 NKJV

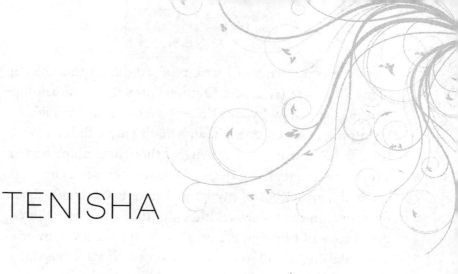

TENISHA

> "It's not whether you get knocked
> down, it's whether you get up."
> — Vince Lombardi

I have learned that God is in control. No matter how much I want to control every aspect of my life, God has the final say. For five years, I tried and tried to get pregnant. I wanted twins so I could get it out of the way. Most certainly a derivative of my Type A personality. I was envious of other women, including Rayan, when I found out they were pregnant with twins. I had to realize that God allows things to happen to show you what's best for you. I cannot carry twins, and if I had gotten pregnant with twins, the likelihood of me carrying was slim to none. I have also learned that my strength extends beyond the physical. My body went through so much but mentally, I had to dig down deep to keep pushing through. My strength also comes from my vulnerability. Being vulnerable allowed me to heal and help others. I'm grateful for the woman I am now.

The worst advice that I have received during this chapter of my life was to try harder. Over and over, it was the assumption that somehow I wasn't doing enough, trying enough, or loving my husband enough, and that's why I didn't have a baby. It was hurtful, and although I thought it didn't bother me, I now realize that it did. It damaged my confidence and chipped away pieces of my hope. I have been wrong about my power in the process. Although often taken for granted, the process of bringing life into the world is truly a miracle and a blessing from God. There are no accidents. Everything happens in God's timing, and I had to accept that it was not my will. I had to relinquish the power to my creator in order to be empowered and focus on my faith.

One thing that I had to unlearn was the lesson that hard work pays off. As a perfectionist, I always believed that I would receive the result I wanted with hard work and persistence. However, after several failed IVF and intrauterine insemination (IUI) cycles and pregnancy losses, I realized that this time was different. My work ethic and "box-checking" weren't going to get the job done. It was about the intangible and immeasurable faith that I needed to get through the journey and get God's promised result. I questioned God repeatedly as to why He gave me this cross to bear.

I have felt lost several times throughout the last five years, especially after each loss. I remember walking into Target and before I could get inside, I started to miscarry in the middle of the road right in front of a police car. The officer asked if I needed an ambulance, and I reluctantly said no because I already knew that it was another loss. My heart sank, and I felt so ashamed and embarrassed. Honestly, I should not have felt these feelings, but I needed a break physically and mentally. It was too much, and I needed to find myself again. I had lost who I was in the shots, ultrasounds, and appointments. I was a robot, and I needed to reclaim myself.

The most challenging part of this phase was its strain on my body. I am forever changed. There are things I can no longer tolerate. I developed allergies that I did not have before, and I gained weight that I couldn't shake off. I knew it was a part of the process and definitely worth it, but it is something that I struggle with now. The best thing about this chapter has been my spiritual growth. I always had a relationship with God, but it was strengthened and transcended during this time. I was able to connect with God on another level, one that I thought only praying grandmothers could achieve. I spoke to God, and God spoke to me. He allowed me to comfort and minister to others despite not having a living child of my own. That level of faith and hope made me a better person. A better wife, daughter, and friend.

However, I regret not grieving long enough after each loss. I realized that grieving is a natural part of loss, and there's nothing wrong with expressing and working through that grief. I did not realize that it would manifest again during what should have been the happiest moment in my life after giving birth to my daughter. Instead of feeling complete joy, I felt guilty about losing my daughters. I started to rehash what I could have done differently to save them instead of remembering that it was not my fault. I had to take a pause and remind myself that I was not in control.

The next chapter that I'm planning to embark on is raising my daughter to be a compassionate and loving person. I want her to be fierce and strong, but also caring and giving. I would love to help other women and families on their journey to parenthood. This is my ministry, and I'm ready to serve others. I know God has given me the ability to speak life to others, and I want to use that gift to help women get through this time and provide them with the financial resources to grow their families. I would continue to try. I would pursue my goal relentlessly until I had achieved my end result. I love talking to strangers about my story. I was always taught to keep your business your business but throughout this journey, I realized that sharing my story has been a blessing to others and myself.

The milestone I'm working toward in my personal life is to be a great mom to my daughter and to pursue having another child. The milestone I'm working toward professionally is to grow my business and legal consulting firm so I can pass it down to my daughter. I believe that I was divinely appointed for this journey because God gives His toughest battles to His strongest soldiers. I feel most alive knowing that the spirits of my daughters and my grandmothers live inside of my baby girl. I would say to myself...be patient because God is working. Your test is for a grand testimony!

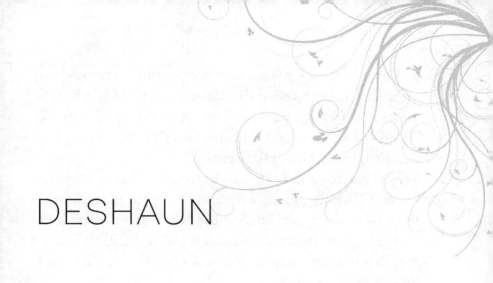

DESHAUN

"We do not attract what we want but what we are."
— James Allen

The lessons in this season of my life are immeasurable. In those moments of perfect peace and reflection, I can find appreciation and honestly say I am grateful—but don't get it twisted. I wouldn't have picked the strife I've had to endure over these past few years. If this was the "road less traveled" and I had a choice in the matter, I am more than confident I'd go the populated route. That said, this is a chapter in my journey of life and although I've bent—and some days truly thought I was broken—I am whole and stronger than ever. I am now fortified with the lessons of timing, gratitude, and perseverance. In life, I was always taught you can achieve anything if you are willing to work for it. Well I am almost certain they left something out of that lesson, and that's God. Despite fasting, praying, diet modification, acupuncture, herbal teas, vitamins from every part of the globe, fertility massages, fertility yoga, timed intercourse, countless shots and blood draws, last-minute trip cancellations because my cycle is starting, meeting disruptions and calendar changes, saints and fertility statues...I can honestly say I/we tried all we knew, researched, and dreamt of but the results just weren't there...yet. While I can't pinpoint a time that this lesson became clear, I can say I learned to relinquish control because I was becoming exhausted trying to control something that I clearly had little control over. I learned that God's timing may not be my timing, but it will be PERFECT timing. This time of trial and tribulation will be reframed as a time of preparation.

I've learned to be grateful during this period of waiting. Now, let's be real. It's not always easy. Sometimes you become so focused on a goal, a dream, a desire, a wish that it starts to consume you without your awareness. One minute you're completely in the moment laughing about foolishness, and the next minute you're on your phone tracking your cycle or keeping an eye on the clock for your next shot. It can be maddening! However, I learned that while I may not have everything I want at this point in my life, I am still blessed and highly favored. I've learned **gratitude** is a choice. You can focus on what you don't have (yet), or you can enjoy what you do have and embrace the wait!

Another key lesson for me was I am stronger than I think. In this journey to motherhood, I lost my grandmother. She was my heart and soul, my confidant, my voice of reason, and my strength. I miscarried twice. I questioned my marriage, and then I lost one of my dearest friends/line sister to breast cancer after a brutal but silent battle. If there is a team for #TooMuch, I'm the captain and the mascot. I have no explanation for how I stood through this, kept it relatively together, and maintained my job, let alone friendships during this time. The minute I started to feel like myself after one hit, life would get sucked out of me again from another hit. If it wasn't the hormones keeping me out of whack, it was the pain and turmoil of indescribable loss. I can compare it to being under water and being able to see the top, but you can't swim up fast enough and you know you're running out of reserved air. Upon reflection, the only reason I survived was because of God. If I think about the poem "Footprints in the Sand" by Mary Stevenson, I am quite sure there is only one set of footprints in this season, and they are the reason I can **persevere**. Again, I wouldn't have elected this struggle, but I've learned if you want something bad enough, you will evaluate all options to make it a reality. What you do during the wait is up to you. A delay is not a denial. *"In their hearts humans plan their course, but the Lord establishes their steps"* – *Proverbs 16:9 NIV*

The term line sister is used to describe women within the same new member class of a historically black greek letter organization.

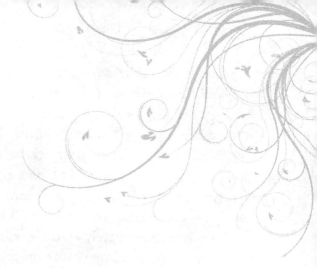

RAYAN

"It is easier to walk on water with faith
than to walk on thin ice with fear."
– Scott Johnson

After settling in a few months following our wedding in June of 2015, I took a home pregnancy test because I felt a little off on the 11th of September.. When the line came back positive, I felt shocked and excited at the same time. The next day, what did I do after seeing the line? I took another one to make sure our blessing was really a reality. And it was so true, we were pregnant. My husband was so excited when he received a picture of those two lines. I could not wait until he returned home to tell him. I wanted him to know at that moment as well. We held this excitement back from the family until we were able to confirm there was an actual heartbeat. I immediately stopped working out because I was too scared due to all the horrible stories I heard. I felt like it would just be my luck to keep working out and experience a devastating event that would make me lose the baby.

At that point, I should have trusted GOD no matter what. I let doubt get the best of me. I went on with my daily routine, so time would pass me by quickly.

I kissed my husband and told him I would see him later when he returned home from work. It was finally time for my first doctor's appointment to put my horrible fears to rest. September 16, 2015, is a day I cannot forget. I was finally ready to see evidence of my dream! I walked into the office, and a nurse immediately escorted me to a room. I was so nervous I could feel the sweat on the palms of my hands. A few minutes later, the doctor entered the room to do an ultrasound to hear the heartbeat and measure our new baby. She walked me through the step-by-step process. She finally advised me to look at the monitor so I could see the unexpected turn. I was not only pregnant with one baby but TWO babies. We could hear and see two heartbeats!!! The doctor named them Twin A & B, and my due date was May 25, 2016. Twin B's heartbeat was only 120 bpm, while Twin A was at 140 bpm. She advised me that 120 bpm was a little low, but the pregnancy was very early so she didn't want me to worry. We would give it about two weeks to see if anything changed. Even though she told me to not worry, I was a nervous wreck. My husband consoled me and kept me positive the entire time. I love that man!

Two weeks later, I was back in the doctor's office to check up on Twin B. After getting in position and watching the screen of my babies, all I could see was Twin B's limp body with no heartbeat. During this heart-crushing time, I could still see Twin A's heartbeat and busy body moving. I had lost Twin B at the six-week mark. Twin A was still measuring a few days ahead and seemed to be doing fine. It was devastation and happiness all at once. My doctor advised me this may have been something called the "Vanishing Twin" syndrome. She thoroughly explained to me that I may pass the baby, or he/she would just deteriorate to make room for Twin A. I had all kinds of mixed emotions at this point. After leaving the doctor's office, all I could do was sit in my car, pray, and cry for my strength but with gratitude that Twin A was doing great. My husband was crushed, but he always has the most encouraging words when setbacks happen.

Let me fast forward to roughly a month later. The morning of November 18, 2015, I started to spot a little, and my head was aching so bad. I remember the doctor telling me the spotting may happen, but I wanted to be safer than sorry. I was in the middle of putting a doctor's visit on my very long to-do list, but a close friend advised me to stop everything and go to the doctor right then. That same day, I made an appointment for the doctor to fit me on her schedule. I arrived at 1:30 p.m. to check on things and ease my fears again. It's just human nature. The doctor performed my ultrasound, and everything was fine. My baby was measuring right on time (13 weeks exactly), and I was even able to record the heartbeat. It was glorious to my ears. I forgot about the horrible headache that was upon me. The doctor and nurse advised me to take Tylenol. Being cautious, I set an appointment to see a neurologist.

A week went by, and I was still spotting and popping Tylenol like crazy for my headaches. On November 27, 2015, I told my husband that I decided to go to the ER that day. Even though we had family in town, I figured I would sneak off to the hospital without them even knowing. When I arrived, the nurse escorted me back to the ultrasound room to check the baby's heartbeat. When I heard no sound and the nurse started acting strange, I knew something was wrong. She advised me that a doctor would need to read my results. By this time, I was nervous and called my husband to join me. They placed me in a room as we waited for the doctor. When the doctor entered and told me that my baby had no heartbeat and had stopped growing at 13 weeks and one day, we were devastated. At the time, mine was supposed to be 14 weeks. All I could think to myself was, "I just left the doctor's office last week, and everything was perfect." The doctor left the room to give us time together to process the heartbreak. All my husband could do was console me because I was crumbling from the news. I had never cried so hard in front of him. I tried to be strong, but my heart would not let me. The doctor returned to advise us of the options I had to pass the baby. She stated we could get a dilation and curettage (D&C) procedure or naturally miscarry the baby. I just wanted the heartache to be over, so I agreed to a D&C. Afterward, they performed the procedure and released me to go home. She told me I may feel some discomfort and pain, but it would be normal.

By this time, my husband had informed the family of what had happened. It felt so awkward when we first arrived home, but they were so loving and supportive of EVERYTHING. I went on with my days as if nothing had happened. Inside, I was very torn apart. With prayer, I was ok.

The days went by, and it was getting closer to the MRI appointment I had set up before my miscarriage. I thought to myself, "You should just skip this appointment because you are now starting to feel better." Something kept bothering me to make my appointment date, so I did and had the MRI on December 23, 2015. I found out I had a large acoustic neuroma tumor on the bottom left side of my brain. The only way to have it removed was surgery. How terrifying was this? But also a blessing because the tumor was non-cancerous.

My surgery was set for the early morning of February 2, 2016. I went through a nine-hour procedure, and the majority of the tumor was removed. The recovery was challenging because I had to learn to re-swallow, re-balance, had limited hearing in my left ear, and needed time to allow my left-side facial paralysis to heal. I am still not 100% from my paralysis, but God is seeing me through the new normal. I thank God for sparing my life because if I knew of all the complications from surgery, it would have been harder for me to endure this setback. I graduated from rehabilitation two months post-surgery, and I also started back doing CrossFit classes at 2.5 months post-surgery. CrossFit helped with my stability tremendously.

HIS Story

"Husbands, love your
wives, just as Christ also
loved the church and
gave Himself for her,"
—Ephesians 5:25 NKJV

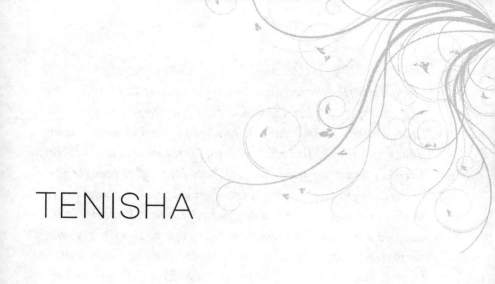

TENISHA

"Where there is love, there is life."

– Unknown

AN INTIMATE INTERVIEW
WITH EVERETTE BROWN

Why did you get married?

Why did I get married? I got married because I love Tenisha. My parents have been married for over 30 years, but I never saw myself getting married unless it was the right person. I wanted to be a father, but I didn't want to be a father outside of marriage. So I guess marriage was inevitable. I knew I wanted to spend my life with Tenisha and in an effort to keep her, I needed to step up and take the leap into marriage. She let me know upfront that even though it was very common for athletes to have kids without being married, which there is nothing wrong with that, she was not interested in being my baby mama and honestly, neither was I.

How would you describe the fertility process?

I would describe the fertility process as unexpected. I had no idea what to expect or that we would even have to go through a fertility process to have a baby. Like most people, I thought having a baby was simple. But after we tried for six months and nothing, Tenisha's doctor suggested we seek help. None of us thought that there was something wrong. In the beginning, everything seemed routine, even when Tenisha had to have surgery. But after losing our first daughter, I was hesitant to try again. Despite my reservations, my wife is Tenisha, and she doesn't take no for an answer. I wasn't hesitant because I didn't want to have a baby. I was hesitant because I saw the hurt and pain that she experienced losing our daughter. It was hard during surgeries, shots, and pills. I just wanted my wife back.

We kept trying but after losing our second daughter, which honestly hurt the most, we both felt like we were done trying. She shut down and blocked everyone out except for me. Everyone called and texted me to see how she was feeling, and it was a lot. When we lost our final IVF baby in 2019 and I watched her face in embarrassment in the Target parking lot, in my mind our process was over. I never wanted to see my wife hurt like that again, and if that meant we would not have a baby, I was ok with that. Looking back now that we have Banx, the process was hard, but I'm glad that we kept trying to get her.

Do men grieve during this process?

Men grieve during this process but in different ways. I didn't feel like I had the space or time to actually grieve. Tenisha was the one feeling the drugs and the losses, so I felt like my time to really grieve was never there. I also didn't realize how losing our daughters affected me. We held both of our daughters, but our second daughter was the one we fought so hard to keep. That one seemed to hurt a little bit more, and I guess it was because we didn't have to use IVF or any other treatment to get her. I would say I managed my grief by focusing on Tenisha and making sure she was ok. I just pushed whatever I was feeling to the side and let her heal.

What challenges did you, personally, face during the process?

The biggest challenge I faced during the process was not having my wife. The process changed her. Her moods, her energy, and just her. Our whole dynamic changed, and I had to figure out how to navigate while she was on medications. When we were high, we were high and when we were low, we were super low. There was no happy medium for five years. Don't get me wrong, I appreciate the process because we are better for it, but that process is hard on you mentally.

What are the other hidden emotions that the husband doesn't often get to express?

I would say the biggest hidden emotions that the husband doesn't get to express are exhaustion and loneliness. Throughout the whole process you are told that you have one job, but that's not true. I had a lot of jobs including being the main support for my wife, which at times was very hard. At some points during our process, I wasn't in the same city because of work. That was tough because I had to figure out how to encourage or console her from far away. When I say exhaustion, I mean I was tired of disappointment. It was exhausting mentally.

As for loneliness, going through this process is very lonely if you don't have anyone to go through it with. None of my friends had experienced this before, and all they could offer was words of encouragement, Honestly they really didn't know what to say. I know they wanted to see us finally become parents, but I never had anyone to really talk to about it.

Who does a man need the most support from?

Most importantly a man needs the most support from his wife, but he also needs an outlet, and that can be a hobby or friends who he can vent to and bounce things off of. The husband needs his "me time" because it can be a heavy situation when you're in it for a long time.

If you could impart some advice to daddy's in waiting, what would that be?

1. *Before you get pregnant and while you're trying to get pregnant, keep the faith and live your life. If you spend every day worrying about it, you will miss so much more that contributes to your beautiful story.*
2. *During pregnancy, I would say work hard to be in tune with your spouse because their body is changing. If you don't, there will be a disconnect between feelings and each other's bodies.*
3. *During pregnancy, be patient and give grace because every day isn't going to be perfect. Every day is a new day, and you have to start fresh and try to win that day.*

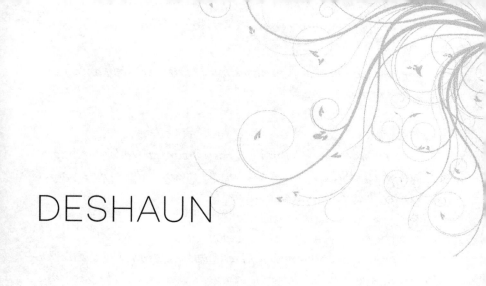

DESHAUN

"You know you're in love when you can't fall asleep
because your reality is better than your dreams."
—Dr. Seuss

AN INTIMATE INTERVIEW
WITH FERNANDO PORTER.

Why did you get married?

*When I graduated from high school, my father had a conversa-
tion with me. The paraphrased version was not to even get a
girlfriend in college, but rather wait until after because I pre-
sumably had the rest of my life to find a mate. As a result of this
advice, what happened was for me to not deny myself a true shot
at finding a lifelong partner. Because of that challenge, I was
so deliberate about love and commitment that when DeShaun
showed the same willingness to be loving and committed to commitment, there was no longer a question about whether or not*

she was "the one." It became a simple matter of when are we get-
ting married?!

How would you describe the fertility process?

As a primary care physician, I have a clinical understanding of
the process. Still, I'm not sure anything can fully prepare you for
the daily emotions accompanying it.

Do men grieve during this process?

The process for everyone is different, but yes. I initially wasn't con-
cerned about failed attempts because I understand the mechanics
of the success and failure rates. But as we continued to face disap-
pointments, the fear of potentially not being able to have children
started to creep in. After the loss of a child through miscarriage,
the most difficult part for me was not being able to grieve together.
The inherent feeling is to be there for your wife, which can ulti-
mately leave you with unresolved emotions. For me, it was
difficult trying to figure out what space you are supposed to be in
to properly grieve. You can't do it at work, your friends probably
don't know, you may not be able to turn to your parents depend-
ing on if they are included or aware. So where do you turn? The
other challenge is while you can get support, unless someone has
experienced a miscarriage before, they don't really understand.

What challenges did you, personally, face during the process?

One of the biggest challenges was not having an outlet to discuss
the process outside of my wife. My wife is a private person, and I
wanted to respect her privacy as she was bearing the brunt of this
process physically.

What are the other hidden emotions that the husband doesn't often get to express?

Not sure if there were hidden emotions, but there is a lack of preparation for what you experience going through the process from a husband's perspective. In most if not all fertility discussions, it is from the female's point of view, but there is a lot that a husband should be informed about at the start of the process. Finding a safe zone to talk about what your wife is going through and how to respond to your wife when she is going through these emotional changes is important because her body is being pumped with hormones, and she may not always be herself.

What support does a husband need amidst this experience?

Agreement from his wife on who (family or friends) can provide support when needed. This may not even mean talking about it in detail, but a safe place/person to go to when we can't go to each other.

Who does a man need the most support from?

Mainly, his wife. Undeniably, this can become a tall order depending on the length of the IVF journey, but a man needs to know he can still turn to his wife even though she is also hurting. The permission and confirmation to hurt together can be helpful.

If you could impart some advice to daddy's in waiting, what would that be?

Here are a few things I would have wanted to know going into the process:

1. *Get your crew together. To put it bluntly, the fertility process was the biggest mind F&%# I've ever experienced, and you're going to need your support system more now than ever. I mean guys who can see you cry, will give you their shoulder to do it on, and will pray for you. You may even want/ need a guy's trip.*

2. *Find your sanctuary. This is the place or activity that you can do alone that brings you joy. You should be able to cry, cuss someone out, think, pray, meditate, or just exist in this space. Mine was cycling.*

3. *Wrap your head around the idea that the person you know now as your spouse/partner will evolve in this process (change temporarily or permanently). This will happen because you are either injecting her with hormones for weeks, months, or years, or because you had a baby.*

4. *Get some understanding about the process and what she will have to go through physically and mentally. It is a long road.*

5. *Plan a trip to either hit reset on your relationship or to celebrate your win in getting pregnant. This will be on you to set the tone on maintaining the relationship through this difficult time, and getting away is a great way to do it. Make it better than your guy's trip and I would recommend more than just one!*

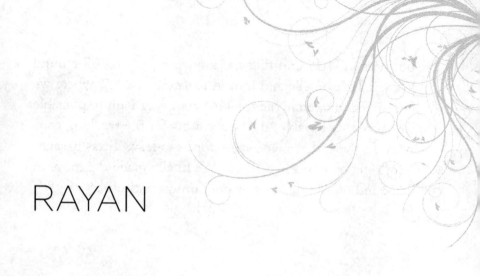

RAYAN

(Through the lens of a wife)

"When someone else's happiness is
your happiness, that is love."

I met my husband in Las Vegas. We occasionally met halfway
with each other and stayed in touch over the years. We tried
to draw away from each other, but faith drew us closer to
one another. In 2014, I moved to Atlanta to be closer to him
because he was in Jacksonville. In 2015, he proposed, and
I moved to Jacksonville. We were married in June of 2015.
Some of the goals we share together as husband and wife are
to be financially stable over a long period of time. One of his
main goals as a husband is to provide for his family.

My main goal is to be able to be there for him and help
to provide for our family. He is a professional athlete who
retired in 2016. His being a professional athlete for us rolled
out perfectly because he was able to walk away from the game
with a sane mindset. We became partners in the trucking

business in 2015 and that trucking company is still around. We left Jacksonville and moved to Texas in 2017, where we continued to operate the trucking company. I am responsible for Accounts Payable, all the accounts for the trucking company. In the end, it made sense for us to leave Texas because our home base was in Atlanta. We finally made the move in 2020 and our desire to grow our family continues.

Freedom and Sharing

"You're braver than you believe, and stronger than you seem, and smarter than you think."
—A.A. Mine

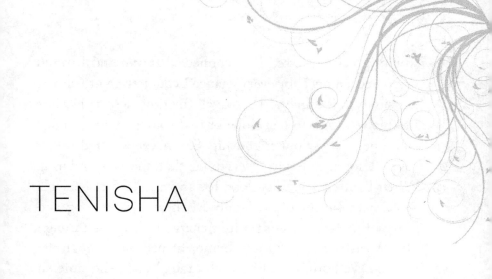

TENISHA

NO NEED TO EXPLAIN,
YOU JUST GET IT

I realized very quickly the power of true friendship during this process, especially friendship with women who know exactly what you are going through. Too often during the journey to motherhood, you feel lonely and isolated. It was a blessing to have individuals in my life who I could intimately share my failures and wins without judgment.

When Rayan and I met, we were both pregnant and due just one day apart. She was pregnant with twins, and I was pregnant with my first daughter conceived through IVF. I wanted twins so badly that I prayed that somehow my singleton would turn into two. She lost the first twin early on and when she was about 13 weeks pregnant, she lost the second twin. As she shared the news with me, I immediately felt her pain and simultaneously felt fear. I never thought about losing a child after the first trimester. We have always been told that if you are going to have a miscarriage, it will happen in the first trimester. Her loss shook me to the core. I would've never guessed how connected Rayan and I would be. I checked my baby every chance I could, trying to ensure her survival. Rayan and I spoke all the time despite her loss. I didn't want her to feel alone or that somehow we couldn't continue to grow our friendship. She never wavered in her support for me despite everything that she was enduring. When I suffered my first loss, Rayan was the first person I spoke with outside of my family. My heart was hurting, and I knew I needed Rayan's positive energy to help me through. Her consistency, loyalty, and humor helped me through the trauma. We both leaned on each other. When she suffered the loss of her daughter, I remember her texting me while she was in the hospital debating on choosing her life over her daughter's. The level of trust we have allows us to be real, raw, and vulnerable. We are forever connected, and I could not imagine this journey without her.

Just as Rayan was my haven, I was called to serve as a haven for DeShaun. I always say that God called me to tell my story and that my journey is my ministry. DeShaun and I have known one another since college. I always admired her because she was the epitome of an Alpha Kappa Alpha woman. I aspired to be like her. When I first met her, I was in awe because she was smart, classy, beautiful, and powerful. Even as we matured as adults, I thought her life was the defi-nition of perfection. I never imagined that she was enduring a similar pain. I couldn't believe that yet another person so close to me was struggling with infertility. Unlike Rayan and me, DeShaun's infertility was unexplained. I felt even more inclined to be there for her just as Rayan was there for me. Even though I was suffering loss after loss, I felt like I needed to be strong for DeShaun. The strength that I found helped me get through every failed trial. As she grieved over failed IVF cycles, I would share with her my stories of successful rounds. I would pray with her and share my successes to keep her spirits up and her hope intact. I did not realize that each call, prayer session, and word of affirmation was not just for DeShaun but also for me. I needed to be there for DeShaun so I could heal as well. God gave her the strength and confidence to share her journey with me in order to help me push through.

LESSON:
FAITH AND
FRIENDSHIP ARE THE
KEY FACTORS IN
GETTING THROUGH
THE STRUGGLE WITH
INFERTILITY.

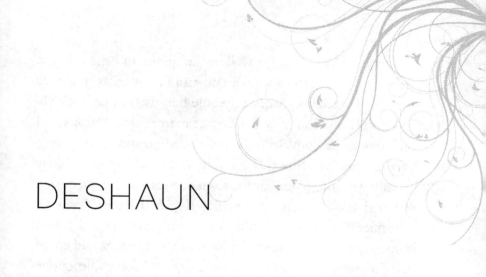

DESHAUN

"Friendship isn't the big thing, it's
a million little things"
—Unknown

Our love for Alpha Kappa Alpha Sorority brought
Tenisha and me together, but it is our life experiences
that formed an unbreakable bond. Since meeting her in the
early 2000s, I can say she has always had a passion for life
and a determination that was unmatched. A prayerful soul
who remained steadfast in her faith despite circumstances,
which bode well as we experienced unexpected challenges on
our journey to motherhood.

I can still recall the day I left a doctor's appointment and
made the decision to call Tenisha to let her know what I
may be facing. Although I knew she was courageous enough
to share her story, I still didn't know if she would be willing to share the difficult details or even headspace to talk
about it, but she was, and she was so gracious. Her optimism
was contagious, and her knowledge of the process was quite

impressive. We talked for well over an hour and she told me everything, from the approximate number of shots to advice on how to make my work schedule because the doctor's visits are endless. This was the first of many conversations and each one more comforting, more uplifting, and more prayerful than the last. She was a haven and privately or publicly encouraged me to be that for someone else in this process.

I had the pleasure of meeting Rayan through Tenisha's introduction, and it was like connecting with an old friend. Immediately we provided the love, support, safety, and space that only another person in your exact position could understand. With both ladies, it was never one big thing but, it was countless little things that would occur JUST as they were needed. Random phone calls, being tagged in a post that offered encouragement, our group chats to make a decision with the choices presented by our doctors—the list is endless but every time, it was right on time!

RAYAN

"Change is inevitable, growth is optional."
Unknown

I met Tenisha through the Professional Football Wives Association (PFWA). We became closer during that time. We became closer throughout meetings and talking to one another, and the relationship became personal. We have been friends ever since. I met DeShaun through Tenisha, and she became our mutual friend. I met her when we first decided to do the book. DeShaun and I also have truly become closer over the years. We talk to each other at least once every two or three weeks. I may text her or she may text me. During her difficult situation, I had encouraging words for her, and she had encouraging words for me when I was going through my own tough times. We keep in touch, and the bond between all three of us is awesome. When we met in Atlanta to do a photoshoot for the cover, that was my first time seeing DeShaun in person, and we just automatically clicked. The greatest value gained from these ladies is true friendship and knowledge because even though our stories are similar, there are differences. Things that I don't know, DeShaun knows. Tenisha has answered some of my questions, and DeShaun has answered some of Tenisha's questions. Friendship and knowledge are the main values gained.

Our Journeys

"But may the God of all grace who called us to His eternal glory by Christ Jesus, after you have suffered a while, perfect, establish, strengthen, and settle you."
—1 Peter 5:10 NKJV

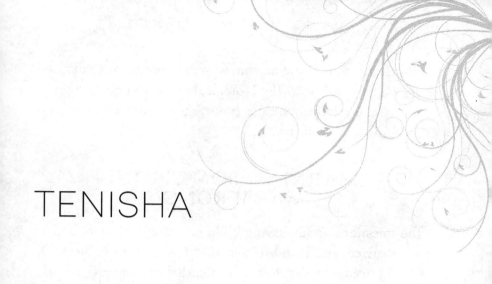

TENISHA

"I can be changed by what happens to
me but I refuse to be reduced by it."
—Dr. Maya Angelou

THE PROCESS

As a woman, regardless of how much you accomplish in your career, there is still the expectation that someday you will bear children or be a mother. There's also an assumption that getting pregnant is easy, and if you don't get pregnant quickly, then that means you're not trying hard enough. Then you have the issue of people constantly asking you when you're going to get pregnant, individuals who are unaware of the fact that you may be having difficulty. Lastly, you have the issue of people looking at you like you have a horrible disease when they find out you are having trouble getting pregnant. The most common question: "What's wrong with you?" Quite frankly, it's grossly insensitive because 99% of the time, it's directed at women. There is a lack of awareness of the emotional state of the person, who may not want to discuss their issues with you. The biological process of getting pregnant seems relatively simple, however, sometimes everything does not work as it should.

LEARNING SOMETHING WAS WRONG

The questions about having children started the moment I got married, and it didn't help that I was about to turn 30. On my wedding day, I was bombarded with questions primarily centered around producing miniature versions of my husband and me. We had been together so long and everyone, especially our parents, were dying to see us have children. We talked about it, but we wanted to wait. We wanted time to enjoy being married but in February 2015, I started a journey that I will never forget.

After nearly three months of reckless behavior with my husband, there were no signs of pregnancy on the horizon. I made an appointment with my gynecologist. I wasn't necessarily trying to get pregnant, but I wasn't preventing it either. After giving me a clean bill of health, she suggested that I go for an hysterosalpingography (HSG) test. She couldn't determine what was going on, but she acted on a hunch. I didn't think anything of it, and I went about my business like nothing was wrong. I went in for my procedure, and I was unpleasantly surprised at how painful it was. I was certainly not prepared. After getting dressed, I waited on my results in the patient area. I only waited for about 10 minutes before the physician's assistant (PA) came over and asked me if I was alone or was my husband in the lobby. I told her I'm alone and immediately asked her what's wrong. Her tone was very somber and somewhat remorseful. At this point, I thought she was about to tell me I was dying. She sat down and began to explain the results of my X-ray. Somehow my fallopian tubes were dilated and blocked, preventing me from getting pregnant. Honestly, even as she was explaining this to me and showing me on my X-rays, I still didn't quite understand why she was so sad. I was just happy she didn't say I had some incurable disease. I was sure she was being overly dramatic, especially after she kept asking me if I was ok. She even had a box of tissues in her hand, just in case. When she finished explaining my results and my next step, she asked if I had any questions, and I said no. She looked puzzled as if she missed something. I reassured her that I didn't have any questions, and I went on my way. I could tell that she was expecting tears, outbursts about how life sucks or why is this happening to me, but I didn't give her that. I was calm, upbeat, and essentially clueless about the severity of my issue.

After leaving my appointment, I still had no idea about the seriousness of my condition. It didn't help that reading an X-ray is nearly impossible for someone who is not in the medical field. I knew it was something that had to be addressed, but I figured it had to be something a pill or two could fix. I didn't bother Googling it because honestly, sometimes the "answers" you find create more anxiety than actual value. I scheduled an appointment with my gynecologist, and her demeanor was more calm than the PA and more of what I expected. She informed me that I needed to see a fertility specialist immediately because it was something that would prevent me from getting pregnant.

After making the decision to pursue IVF, I was immediately bombarded with questions and concerns by family and friends. Questions surrounding the nature of the procedure, because they had no idea how it would actually work, and concerns about my safety. IVF is tough on your body, especially following a surgery that requires time to heal. Unfortunately, IVF is a bed of artificial stimulation. As my doctor explained the process of IVF and how the medications replace the natural process that your body goes through, I found myself in awe at the greatness of God. It takes so much just to imitate the natural processes of creating life, something that I had taken for granted for so many years. I knew there would be several medications, but I wasn't prepared for the package I received. As I opened the box and pulled out medication after medication, I couldn't believe that my name was actually on every single one. From pills to injections that required me to do far more than I could have imagined, I was dumbfounded. I was immediately overwhelmed and anxious about messing it up. I called my best friends, who are PAs, and demanded that they move in with me so they could give me my injections. I realized that I was being a little dramatic. Obviously, they said no and insisted that I was more than capable of doing it myself.

As I contemplated whether I was going to actually go through with this, I decided to call my grandmother, my faithful prayer warrior. She didn't quite understand the IVF process, however, she understood that when God is leading you in a direction, you must listen and trust that He will give you the strength to get through your challenges. As I described to her the amount of pills I would have to take and the type of injections, I instantly felt foolish. I was complaining about something I prayed for, something that was necessary to become a mother, and something that was so miniscule compared to what she goes through on a daily basis. I reminded myself that she knows about all these things. She knows about injections because she must endure dialysis. She knows about multiple pills because she must take them on schedule daily. One fact remained true, she never complained. Without even a lecture, she snapped me back to reality. I asked for this. I wanted this. I was blessed with this. So I chose to put on my big-girl panties and be positive.

PROCESSING THE DISAPPOINTMENT

On December 16th, I began to feel sharp pains in my abdomen. I couldn't figure out what it was and after two hours of suffering, I called for my husband to take me to the hospital. I could barely make it down the stairs due to the pain. We finally made it to the car and right before I got in, my water broke. I couldn't control my emotions. I wanted to fall to the ground, but my husband caught me. He carried me in the house and he immediately called 911. The ambulance arrived, but I knew it was already too late. At 17 weeks, the likelihood of baby Mackenzie surviving was virtually impossible. There was no rush to the hospital. The ride was slow and even after we arrived at the ER, there was no mad dash to save her. I lost all of my amniotic fluid and although she still had a heartbeat, we all knew it was the end. Due to her size, I had to deliver her, which took almost 24 hours of labor. Mackenzie Grace was born at

9:36 p.m. on December 17, 2015. She was a beautiful baby girl, and she looked just like her daddy. Just before midnight, we said our last goodbyes to our baby girl. Losing her is the hardest thing I have ever experienced in my entire life. Thoughts of doubt and fear rushed through my mind as I held her in my arms. How could God bless me with this beautiful little girl and then take her away from me? What could I have done to prevent this? I felt my faith slipping. I couldn't process what was going on and the more I thought about it, the more tears began to flow. I felt her spirit, and I have faith that she's our little angel. As I began to grieve, I was compelled to write. I had intentions of posting a blog on the morning I lost Mackenzie Grace announcing her pending arrival, but God had other plans. I didn't know why this happened, but I knew that the only way I could get through this was through prayer.

ACCEPTING THAT I MAY NEVER KNOW WHY THIS HAPPENED

For months, I endured tests and exams trying to figure out what went wrong. I went from one specialist to another, and no one could find anything. My daughter was perfectly healthy, and so was I. Naturally, this bothered me. How could this be? If there is nothing wrong with me or with my daughter, then why did this happen? I pondered this question repeatedly until one night when I read this scripture: *"Trust in the Lord with all your heart and lean not on your own understanding; in all your ways submit to him, and he will make your paths straight."* Proverbs 3:5-6 NIV. I realized there are some things that I will never understand and that the only solution is to trust that God is in control and knows exactly what He is doing. My hope for my journey to motherhood is welded in my faith and trust in God's will.

REALIZING THAT I WILL NEVER "GET OVER IT."

As I planned for my grieving process—yes, I attempted to plan my mourning—I rationed out time that I would spend grieving before I "got over it." Every time I thought that I was over it, those feelings of hurt came rushing back, and I would break down in tears. I didn't realize that I will never "get over it." Yes, I will heal, but it wasn't healthy or productive to spend time trying to forget what happened. I will never forget how I felt about my daughter or how I felt the night I lost her, however, I will heal. I learned that losing a child isn't something you "get over," and no one expects that of you. I had to be patient with myself and with the process. I decided to put all the letters, messages, and cards that I received in a special box along with her angel blanket and booties to honor her. I still have moments of sorrow but in those times, I find solace in my faith.

My journey to motherhood has not been perfect or even ideal, however, I would not trade my experience for anything in the world. This was my test so I can have a testimony!

COPING WITH REGRET GUILT, AND ANXIETY

The realities of struggling with infertility include a certain level of anxiety and guilt. The anxiety is deafening and isolating. I had to consistently remind myself that God is in control. After each transfer, I would hold my breath hoping and praying that this time would be different. After three failed IUIs, four failed IVF cycles, two losses in the first trimester, two losses in the second trimester and five surgeries, my anxiety level was off the charts. The anxiety was turning into insecurity and filtering over in other aspects of my life. I began to question myself in business and my legal career.

Although in most cases I could push through, my trigger was a baby shower. One of the first things that you are told when you struggle with infertility is to avoid circumstances that force you to deal with the realities of your struggle. Some women struggle with seeing other pregnant women or spending time with newborns, but none of that bothered me. However, baby showers gave me a level of anxiety that took my breath away. I avoided every single baby shower invitation until I was forced to celebrate my best friend and her bundle of joy.

When she shared with me that she was pregnant, I was overjoyed because I knew she would be an amazing mother, but I was also disappointed that she didn't feel comfortable sharing her pregnancy struggles with me. She had been struggling with complications that threatened the viability with her pregnancy, and I had no idea she was even pregnant. Immediately following the joy of knowing that my best friend (my sister) was going to be a mom, I felt a sense of loneliness and guilt. I wondered if sharing my story and being so open about my journey was my open display of a scarlet letter. As my best friend cried on my shoulder with fear in her eyes about possibly losing her baby girl, I spoke words of affirmation and faith over her. We prayed for healing in the bathroom stall during our friend's wedding rehearsal. Every word that flowed from my mouth poured from my heart as I petitioned God on her behalf. We stood there in tears thanking Him in advance for the blessing of saving her unborn child's life. I knew exactly how she was feeling, and it is a feeling I would not wish on anyone. That prayer was the same prayer I prayed when I lost my daughters.

God heard our prayers and kept her little angel safely in her womb. As she progressed in her pregnancy, I wanted to share in every moment, but my heart was heavy. I began to avoid her, missing calls and refusing to engage in conversations about the highs and lows of pregnancy. I was having a tough time, and I was disappointed in myself. I felt guilty that I wasn't there for my best friend, but I felt even more guilt that I couldn't carry a child. I knew that my levels of anxiety and guilt would increase if I attended her baby shower that I was also hosting along with our two other best friends. Praise God for their understanding and patience for helping me get through the planning process. I contemplated not attending, but I knew that my fears and anxiety were not worth ruining 20 years of friendship. After months of self-inflicted pressure, it was finally time for the shower. I drove nine hours straight, and I prayed the entire time. I needed God to get me through the day without shedding tears for my angel babies. The moment I walked in the door, my heart stopped. The room was beautifully decorated and overwhelmingly baby. Flashes of my births and losses filled my mind, and I rushed to the bathroom before anyone could see my face. I knew I could not hide in the bathroom for long, so I was forced to pull myself together. I said my prayer and then God sent me my angels.

My best friends and my sorority sisters took my cross and carried it for me.

On that day, a weight was lifted. The fear, anxiety, and guilt seemed to fade away, and I felt renewed in my journey. I needed to face my fear and be reminded that faith and fear cannot coexist. I left the baby shower with a feeling of gratitude. God pulled me through what I believed would be my downfall. It was also reaffirmed that my time would come. Sometimes we create our own anxiety by establishing mental barriers that prevent us from healing.

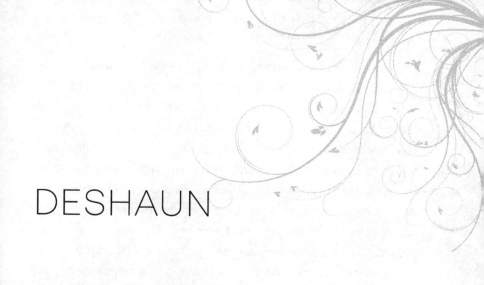

DESHAUN

"When you face difficult times, know that
challenges are not sent to destroy you, they're
sent to promote, increase and strengthen you."
– Unknown

THE PROCESS—
UNEXPLAINED INFERTILITY

Receiving your first IVF medication shipment can be a jar-
ring experience. Needles, sharp containers, alcohol swabs,
meds that you can't pronounce, needles, needles, and more
needles. I consider myself to be one of the fortunate ones
who is married to a doctor, so I didn't have to watch the
how-to videos and build up the courage to administer the
shots to myself, but reality set in just looking at the box
of meds. From there is the monitoring. When you start a
cycle, you go in for monitoring, on average, every other day.
Balancing work and multiple doctor's appointments a week
is stressful, but there is also an emotional experience at every

visit due to the unknown. In my case, I was initially given the diagnosis of unexplained infertility, which later progressed into diminished ovarian reserve (DOR), but more on that later. At the monitoring appointments, you go in praying that your follicles are developing, your lining is thick, and your hormone levels are rising appropriately. The variables under consideration are endless. All the while you are on your way to work, so you don't even have the time to give way to the emotions you are feeling. There you are. Waiting, praying, taking your meds, going to your visits, trying to eat right, exercise, and trying to stay sane–all in hopes of achieving your heart's desires. Your follicles increase in size, you gain some and you lose some in the process. Every measurement and follicle count matters. Then finally, Yay! You make it to egg-retrieval day. Now the eggs can be extracted from your body, mixed with the sperm, and transferred back to you in a couple of days. "Thank God for modern medicine!" The process is quick–you hardly remember it because they knock you out--and you spend the day resting. The emotion experienced here? Hope.

Hope travels with you to one of the days you have been waiting for. Transfer day! You made it, with day-five embryos! The emotion of hope is accompanied with happiness and consumes you, and yet you are still fighting down every negative thought of failure that may cross your mind. You fight off those thoughts as you go through what becomes the agonizing two-week wait. Every blog will tell you don't dwell on it and for the most part, I didn't. I prayed and prayed and prayed some more, but I can say that during this time, I noticed EVERY SINGLE TWINGE in my body and prayed that it was all due to implantation.

Unfortunately my first time around was unsuccessful, and my heart sank. My very first thought was *"How am I going to break this to my husband? He's been such a trooper."* I think I hurt more from the thought of having to disappoint him than I did from the fact that it didn't work, but God hadn't forsaken me. We received a positive pregnancy test on our second transfer. We were simply overjoyed. Honestly, the thought of anything going awry never crossed my mind but alas, we stumbled across the one who comes to steal, kill, and destroy—the devil. A few weeks shy of the second trimester, we were informed that the baby wasn't developing and that-the pregnancy would likely end in a miscarriage. I could hear my heartbeat over the doctor's words. It was almost deafening. I could feel the tears swelling in my eyes and could almost hear each tear as it rolled down my cheek and onto the floor. I can only assume the visit ended with some words of hope but who cared, I was devastated.

I can recall leaving the office with my husband, but I don't remember the words that were exchanged. We both needed time to process, but oh, duty calls. My husband walked me to my car, then to his and went to work. I, on the other hand, must have been on autopilot because I am not sure I was in a state to drive, but I did. I drove to the airport and boarded my plane to Europe for work. (Crazy huh? I know. We will explore this later!) Sitting at my gate waiting to board, I had two emotions: Anger and disbelief. I was angry because how could we come this far and end up with this news? *Had God abandoned us? Did He not hear my prayers, which were now more like pleas?* The disbelief was because we transferred a grade-A embryo (yes, your embryos get grades based on quality), so why would it not survive? It seemed unfair.

While in the UK, I started bleeding. The miscarriage was happening and no amount of prayer, money, or denial was going to stop it. My strength was waning. I needed time to process and heal.

PROCESSING THE DISAPPOINTMENT

For a long time, I felt an unquenchable sense of abandonment and loneliness. Not because of my two angel babies or the loss of my grandmother, or the loss of my dear friend/line sister, but because I felt abandoned by God. I just could not fathom how I had tried to do so many things right in life just to be dealt this hand. Like, how could this happen? I was able to achieve success in so many areas of my life, but the more I longed for motherhood, the harder the struggle became. Clearly, this is not fair. Actually, it's borderline ridiculous and cruel. Who would put their child through this? The harder I prayed, the more bad news I would get from the doctor. It just didn't make sense. I would cry, scream, and sometimes I was downright angry, but there was ALWAYS a calm after the storm. I would get a sense of peace that can't be explained, and then I'd get a rush of adrenaline that would allow me to regroup and devise a plan to try again. That would be followed by a sense of courage and hope, then a small whisper: *"It will happen, just believe."* So have I been wrong? HECK YES! God never abandoned me. He's been with me the whole time and in my lowest moments, clearly it was Him who carried me.

UNSOLICITED ADVICE

If only I had a dollar for every time someone told me "Don't worry about it." This unsolicited piece of advice I was often given would have given me enough money to fund two IVF cycles out of pocket without insurance. LOL. Now on the surface, the advice isn't horrible. In fact, many couples get pregnant the minute they stop "trying" (clocking ovulation, timed intercourse, watching the moon, etc.) or get ready to start fertility treatments. But the advice is out of line and ill-informed. For starters, the audacity of anyone to tell someone to not worry about the very thing you've turned their life upside down to accomplish. It's like telling a small business owner who mortgaged their property and borrowed against their 401K to not worry about their business being closed for months due to COVID. It's just insensitive, and there is a high probability that your four words of advice were unsolicited. At the time one is even ready to share that getting pregnant isn't easy, it's very likely that their struggle didn't start last month. Advice like this in many cases may be harmless and good intentioned, but if it is ill-informed . Be ok with the pregnant pause of silence and stay silent. Pun intended! "You have plenty of time." Studies show that women are having babies well into their 40s now with no problem, and for the stars, their 50s! However, there are women in their 20s who are declared infertile. The truth is, studies are good at educating you on the "average," but how many of us are average?

Every cycle is unique and every body is unique. Unless someone is looking at your medical records, this is an unin-formed statement that can cause a downward cycle for that aspiring mother. Note: Even doctors make this statement and get it wrong.

RELINQUISHING CONTROL

In this experience, I've had to unlearn that if I work hard, I can accomplish anything. A life is a gift from God so while I must do my part–eat well, stay in shape, get rest–God is in charge. The shallow part of me wants to know why it is so easy for someone who relies on government assistance by choice or someone who is abusing or neglecting their child to have multiple children. But there are others who followed the Good Book–independent, waited for marriage to have children, etc.--and they struggle. I'm going to steer clear of questioning God on that one. So, I would like to understand why certain tests are not performed during your OB/GYN appointments, such as testing your anti-müllerian hormone (AMH). It's a simple test that can be an indicator of fertility, but it's not given regularly.

I definitely felt lost in my path many times, heck I may feel lost tomorrow, but the good thing is it doesn't last long. On this journey, it is easy to feel lost. Eventually I realized that while I long for motherhood, it will come as an addendum to my life and perhaps not my sole purpose, so I try to focus on things that bring me joy. If I'm really down, I focus on things that come easy and will give me quick wins to get me going again. I try to not dabble in regrets but if I had a do-over, I would have frozen my eggs at a younger age when I realized it was unlikely that I'd be married by 30 having ended a relationship shortly before marking that birthday.. Also, I wouldn't have canceled ANY of my scheduled trips for a cycle. I love to travel, no I LIVE to travel, and both my husband and I canceled really important trips because of doctor's appointments, meds, etc. Within reason and in retrospect, I would have just lived life. This too will come to pass in God's timing, not mine.

The most challenging thing about this journey is learning to relinquish control. Before this experience, I had no clue that I was somewhat of a control freak. I learned that I am much more relaxed when I have control of a situation, or at least, exiting a situation. For example, I initally didn't realize the reason why I always like to drive my car to the club or an outing is because when I am ready to go, I want to be in full control of my exit and its timing. Unfortunately during this journey, there are so many things within my control—my diet, taking my meds on time, etc.--but the one thing that I have absolutely no control over is the outcome. How humbling. The revelation here was things in and out of my so-called control, I really didn't have control at all. God is the Alpha and the Omega, I'm just along for the ride.

Another challenging thing was deciding when enough was enough. Through poking and prodding, needles, weight loss/gain, doctor's appointments four times a week and mood swings, you can lose your whole self in this process. There were days, weeks, and months that I was literally a shell of myself. I couldn't recognize myself. My loved ones gave me love and grace, but I rejected it because it just felt like pity. Despite the advice, I needed a break. I needed to find me, or the new me because after an experience like this, it's impossible to come out the same person. You can only hope and pray that you come out better than you were before.

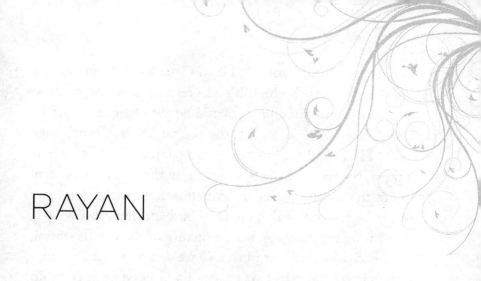

RAYAN

"The rewards for those who persevere far exceed
the pain that must precede the victory."
– Ted W. Engstorm

THE PROCESS: *2ND PREGNANCY*

I had just returned on November 9th from my husband's game and celebrating my birthday two days earlier with my best friend. Something felt a little off with my body. I figured taking a pregnancy test would not harm anything. Low and behold, the test came back positive. The line was very faint, so I decided to wait two more days before taking another one. I thought to myself, "Has God answered my prayer?" After losing the first pregnancy and discovering the brain tumor, I immediately knew this was a blessing I wanted to experience with my husband—all the happy milestones, gender reveal, baby shower, and maternity pictures, cheesy belly progress pictures, etc. After brain surgery, we also discovered I had high blood pressure. I told myself I was not going to get excited until I confirmed it was true I was pregnant and I had confirmed the high blood pressure could be manageable during my time of joy. I waited two long days before taking another test. Again, the pregnancy test came back POSITIVE, and the line was getting darker. To see that plus sign on the test was the best feeling in the world. After staring at the test for about five minutes, I started crying tears of joy. I could not wait to tell my husband the great news. I sent him a text message with a picture of the results stating God had answered our prayer. Once again, we had another little one on the way. I was excited and nervous once again because all the fear kept entering my mind. I immediately set up a doctor's appointment to confirm what I knew and to verify this was a viable pregnancy.

My appointment was set for the morning of November 14. It was football season, I kissed my husband as he headed off to work, and I headed off to my doctor's appointment. I was so nervous when the doctor entered the room. They had me take a urine pregnancy test when I first arrived, so I knew she was coming in to give me my results. She confirmed that I was very pregnant, and we would set up another appointment for an ultrasound on November 30. Was God blessing us for real this time? Did he know my heart's desire? All of these questions were running through my head when I left that appointment. Of course, my husband was so excited, but we decided we would not tell anyone at this time. That was the hardest secret of my life. While waiting for my doctor's appointment to come, I also set an appointment with my internal medicine doctor. He was able to see me immediately. He explained to me that he had previously put me on high blood pressure medication that would not affect my unborn child had I become pregnant again. This was music to my ears! He just advised us to watch things closely and go from there. He sent my labs over to my other doctor so they could adjust my dosage as needed. I thought I was definitely on top of things this time, and things were off to a good start.

The morning of November 30 finally came, and it was time for my ultrasound. As I waited, I patiently prayed for everything to be fine. I felt like everything was in slow motion at this point. Once she started my ultrasound and I saw this tiny little miracle with a heartbeat, my heart smiled. I didn't want to stop watching. It was a viable pregnancy, and baby Marks had a strong heartbeat. I felt a sense of happiness again! My due date was set for July 24.

Through the weeks, I went through many rollercoaster moments because of Google. I finally prayed about it and decided to live my life with happy moments vs. worry. I felt if anything was to happen during this pregnancy, I wanted to be able to relive the greatest moments. I took many pregnancy progress pictures that I shared with my family and close friends. I was determined to continue working out, nothing strenuous, and continue my day-to-day life as we waited on our miracle.

At 16 weeks, I was getting ready to go out of town for the weekend and knew I would be photographed in several pictures, so I happily made the announcement on social media that we were expecting a baby girl. We were experiencing the most precious time of our lives because a baby girl was now showing to the world. The Lord knows I sometimes worry too much, but I felt my worries that were left go out the window. Throughout the weeks, I attended consistent check-ups, high-risk appointments, and numerous ultrasounds. We wanted to make sure we did everything we could to make this pregnancy go smoothly. It was the best experience to start feeling my baby girl kick.

I was 21 weeks and five days into my pregnancy. On March 16, I had a regular doctor's appointment. I had not been to an appointment in a whole month. What I thought was a normal day became a nightmare. The nurse began my appointment by taking my weight. In one month, I went from 154 lbs. to 175 lbs. That was the beginning of the red flags. Next she took my blood pressure, and it was beyond high. Lastly she tested for protein in my urine, and the results sky-rocked, which was not good at all. She advised me to immediately go to labor and deliver. I didn't know what to think. I called my husband and advised him I was going to the hospital, and I would call him as soon as I found out more information. I could hear that he was terrified, so I assured him everything would be ok. I was just going for a routine visit, and they would get my blood pressure under control. Well by the time I was at the hospital and admitted, my blood pressure was close to stroke level. They immediately started magnesium in my IV. The medicine made me so sick that everything I had eaten earlier that day came up. I felt horrible from throwing up multiple times. All I could drink was water to stay hydrated, which was when they found out that I had a severe case of pre-eclampsia and my kidneys were failing. They also told me that because of my severe condition, we would have to deliver my pre-term baby. My heart totally dropped out of my body. At this point, I was totally devastated. I had remained calm the whole time, but the news I received was like ripping my heart out. I hadn't cried so hard since my first pregnancy failed.

At this point, I was in denial and refusing to accept the only option I had. I asked the doctor what would happen if I continued the pregnancy, and she explained a long list of issues, including death. I could feel my husband staring at me with fear in his eyes. By this time, the doctor had left so my husband and I could have a moment alone. I knew he was hurting, but he is one of the strongest men I know. He immediately looked at me and said, "I know we want this baby and would do anything to keep her, but I don't know what I would do without you." Immediately, I fell apart!!! I felt like I had to choose life between my baby and me. God knows the decision I wanted to make. After about an hour of having a moment with my husband, I decided I had to stay here for him, but Lord knows that was the hardest decision of my life.

On March 18, 2017, at 7:44 a.m., I gave birth to a baby girl weighing 9 oz. named Rylee Naomi Marks. Not only did I just give birth, but I naturally pushed out my sweet angel. She was premature. There was nothing the doctors could do for her to make it here on earth. My sweet Rylee passed away two hours later. The caring nurses made sure I had pictures of her. This is a day in my life I will never forget, and sometimes find myself still grieving over my sweet love child. No one can ever be prepared to make funeral arrangements for their child, but by the grace of God, I was able to push through.

On March 31, Rylee Marks was cremated and placed into a small, heart-shaped box. I always hold that tiny box near my heart. To this day, my sweet angel sits amongst her daddy and me in our bedroom, and I talk to her all the time. Her father is my heartbeat on earth, but the love for my angel child has never changed. I cannot thank God enough for giving me the strength to get through and continuing to help me be strong. True enough, I do have some bad days, but the love He has for me lets me cleanse my tears and keep moving. You will never know the feeling of losing a child until it happens to you. I still wonder to this day if God would have performed a miracle had I chosen the other route. I cannot keep dwelling on the past, but I thank God for keeping me on this earth to figure out my purpose.

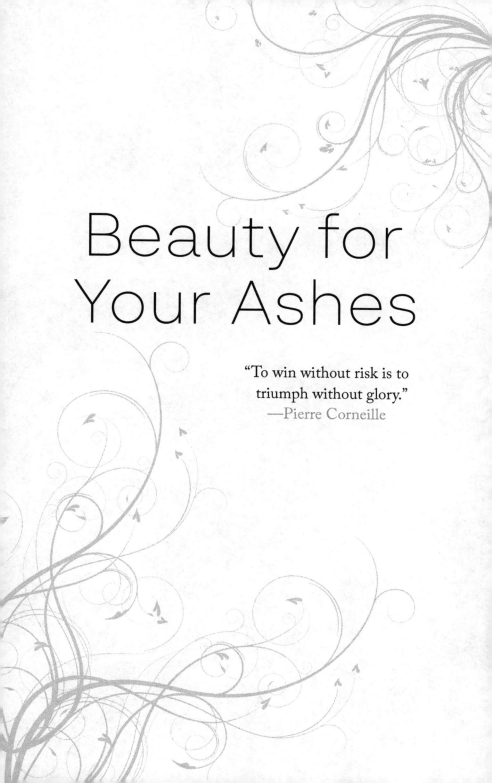

Beauty for Your Ashes

"To win without risk is to
triumph without glory."
—Pierre Corneille

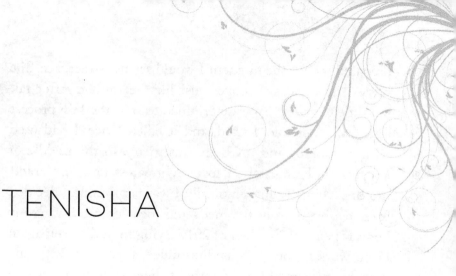

TENISHA

"Blessed is the one who perseveres under trial
because, having stood the test, that person
will receive the crown of life that the Lord
has promised to those who love him."
—James 1:12 NIV

The constant theme that has resonated throughout my life has been positive vibes only. My grandmother instilled in me at a very young age that you can only control how you react and not what happens to you. So, I insisted on having a positive outlook on my life. There is no need to dwell on what could have been or plans falling through because none of that can be changed. This remained true as my husband and I endured through our journey to becoming parents. After losing our daughter, I was sure that the worst was over. I needed time to recover, but I was positive that losing her was my one trial and my testimony was just around the corner.

Losing my daughter in my second trimester meant that I had to go through labor and delivery. Nothing could have prepared me for the moment I would see her sweet face. She was so tiny, and she looked just like her father. After taking time to grieve, I was determined to start the IVF process as soon as possible. I tried, and it failed twice. I had used all my embryos and my body was weary. In the middle of my final IVF transfers, I lost my greatest love, my grandmother. Mentally and physically, I was tapped out. I decided to take a break from the meds and focus on reclaiming my body. I spent the first half of 2017 trying to find myself again. From working out to spending much needed quality time with my husband, I finally started to get back into my groove. When I found out I was pregnant in 2017, it was the classic case of I didn't know I was pregnant. I started the IVF process again and began to take meds. I had no idea that I was already pregnant. I started to have a strange reaction to the meds, and I immediately decided to take a pregnancy test. I was pregnant and despite the 1% chance, my daughter Madison Grace was conceived naturally. I was elated, and I truly believed the worst was behind me. Positive vibes only! Once I approached week 16 of my pregnancy, I began to pray a little harder. When I made it to week 17, I just knew in my heart that my struggle was over. At exactly 18 weeks pregnant, I went into labor and gave birth to my second daughter. As I laid in the hospital bed, I prayed and prayed for God to save my baby. I was angry that God would allow this to happen to me a second time, but I still believed that my daughter would be saved. Unfortunately, despite my pleas and willingness to risk my own life to save hers, my angel was called home. I was devastated. Emotionally and physically drained. I wanted to mask the pain so once again, I threw myself into IUI and IVF cycles that were destined to fail.

I spent all of 2018 trying to get pregnant. Each month I would try, and each month I would be disappointed. In November of 2018, I found out I was pregnant again but right after Thanksgiving, I had another miscarriage. I wanted to try one more time using our last embryo. In December 2018, I had a successful IVF transfer, and I was pregnant. Unfortunately, once again my hopes were met with disappointment. I had a false pregnancy. My body thought I was pregnant, but there was no baby. I decided not to have a D&C, but I was not prepared for the trauma of profusely bleeding in the middle of the Target parking lot. I was embarrassed and ashamed. Most notably, I was done. I felt like I was tapped out, and I simply couldn't do it anymore. I was tired of trying to get pregnant with children I felt I was destined to lose.

After loss after loss, I decided once again that it was time for me to heal. I needed to focus on my mind and body without trying to get pregnant. I started a full detox including removing meat from my diet. My days consisted of working out, meditation, and overall living my best life. I wanted to love myself and my husband. We had spent the last five years of our lives in baby mode, and it was time for us to enjoy ourselves. Although I had never carried a child full-term, I knew in my heart that one day I would be a mother again. So I shifted my focus away from getting pregnant, and we asked our family and friends to avoid the subject. We didn't want to feel the pressure of reproducing or discussing where we were in the process. After eight months of self-care, God sent me two angels. Two of my fellow NFL sisters offered the greatest gift you could offer someone in my position. They offered to be my surrogate. As they spoke those words, they both proclaimed that God put it on their hearts and offered their wombs. It was a beautiful expression of love and honestly, I will never forget the gratitude that I felt in those moments. God never puts more on you than you can bear. His plan is greater than ours, and sometimes we must endure to reap the grand blessing.

FAITH OVER FEAR: REMEMBERING GOD'S PROMISE

"I will look on you with favor and make
you fruitful and increase your number, and
I will keep my covenant with you."
—Leviticus 26:9 NIV

Throughout my journey to motherhood, my mantra was that God always keeps His promises. I believed in my heart that God would not leave me and that all my struggles would be rewarded. I talked to God, and I knew that my timing was not His timing. There were lessons that had to be learned throughout this process, lessons that would take time and ultimately make me the woman and mother God needed me to be. Each time I suffered a loss, I dug deeper into the Word. I found myself connecting with Job. I felt that if Job, who was stripped of everything and still maintained his faith, was rewarded for his faithfulness, then so would I. So I prayed and prayed. There were moments that I doubted. I was angry with God because I could not understand why He would bless me with a successful pregnancy and then take that child away from me. But every time my faith would waver, I would be reminded of the blessings in my life. God never said no, He just said not right now. God always keeps his promises!

I did not give up on my journey to motherhood, but I did recognize that this journey is not a sprint. Being strong doesn't always mean you keep going even when you are tired. Sometimes true strength is recognizing when you need to rest. With patience, self-care, and most importantly faith, I was confident I would be a mother again. By God's grace, I was right. Every trial led to a grand testimony. After six years of losses, struggles, and 1% chance conversations, my baby girl Banx Elyse Brown was born after natural conception. The joy I felt carrying a healthy baby was beyond words. Each day I look at her face, I'm reminded that God always keeps His promises!

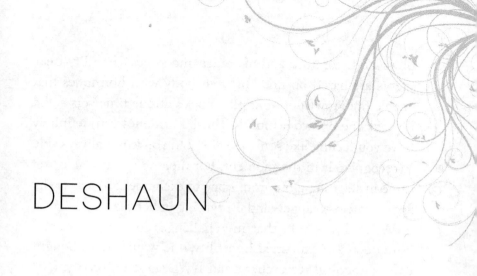

DESHAUN

"You were given this life because
you're strong enough to live it."
—Unknown

Women who end up having a less than smooth path to motherhood will be most impacted. However, I strongly believe sisters, mothers, and friends can all benefit from learning about the struggles so they can provide support and encouragement to their loved ones if needed. When I think about how many people are impacted by this struggle compared to how often it is discussed, it is heartbreaking to know that so many of us suffer in silence and deal with feelings of inadequacy with little support or real understanding of the pain. The emptiness can be equated to the deafening silence while being in a room full of people.

The journey to motherhood through fertility treatments is EMOTIONAL. If you think about it logically, many women experience PMS, which is naturally mood-altering and can cause fluctuations in body temperature, change in eating habits, physical discomfort, and of course, moodiness. Fertility treatments are based on flooding your body with hormones that enable the growth of multiple follicles at one time versus the normal one or two a month. Those hormones can definitely leave you feeling like someone else, and you're not always able to recognize it in the moment. For me, the emotional aspect came in stages ranging from hope to excitement to fear to disappointment to anger—and everything in between.

When I was told that my challenges in bearing a child were due to unexplained infertility, one would have thought I was a medical researcher at an Ivy League university. I sat for countless hours with medical books, dictionaries, "fertility" recipes, white papers, and Google opened across 10-plus tabs on my laptop either defining a term or breaking down the statistical significance of different studies. Of all the podcasts, quotes, or articles, the ones I found to be most helpful were the stories/blogs from others going through similar challenges. These were most meaningful not because they confirmed a specific protocol or shared the side effects that the doctors forget to tell you, but because they provided hope. Thousands of women flock to blogs during this time, not because it is going to give them the proper protocol but because it is a safe place to share your concerns without being judged or told to not worry about it. These forums give you courage when you've tapped out, hope when you've had another canceled cycle, and peace of mind when you think you're losing it.

"Really God, this is my battle/burden? Ok, this is surreal, but let's do this!" Naturally, I had questions as to why I/we were chosen for this battle, but I also had strong confidence that we would have success in the first round.

My (our) journey is our own. While we can't expect others who are not on this journey to fully understand and appreciate all the ups and downs to these tribulations, I want my readers (my extended family) to know that I do. Read my story and pull from it solace knowing that you are not alone, courage to keep trying through the brokenness and despair, and faith to keep you focused that His promises will prevail. There is unbelievable pain in my stories–both physical and emotional–but the journey is one of courage, faith and "soon to be" triumph.

LIFE HAPPENS & THE JOURNEY CONTINUES....

"Please hurry, I'd like to meet my great grandchild and I don't know how much longer I can hold on." *Heart drops* My centenarian? grandmother said those words in the meekest, warmest voice. This was not to apply pressure or evoke depression, but to literally put it in the atmosphere that it was her wish. In July 2019, I started another cycle, but would you believe after the pokes and prodding, endless doctor's appointments, chiropractors, acupuncturists, and fertility teas–to name a few–my body wouldn't respond to the meds. Cycle canceled. I wish I could tell you I was mad, but that would probably be an understatement. In August, I watched my grandmother's health decline. I felt helpless, like I just knew God would somehow have her pull through until I had a baby, but that was a fleeing thought because this wasn't about me. She was in pain. I listened to her tell stories of her talking to her best friend, Aunt Lou, and my grandfather–both of whom were deceased for years–and I cried. I've never had to do life without my best friend, my confidence, my No. 1, my teacher, my coach, my everything—so I vacillated from holding out hope to praying for strength.

On September 21, we celebrated her birthday. On September 23, I had a tough decision to make: Go to San Diego for work or stand vigil over my grandmother, who seemed to be comfortable but not really responsive. She hadn't eaten for four days, wasn't drinking water, and hadn't urinated in several hours. While my dad tried to hide it, the home nurses couldn't get their story straight. I knew something was wrong, but also knew this was out of my hands. Again, she was in pain. Hours before my flight, I packed my bags and headed to her house. I talked. I think she listened. I cried, she fidgeted. Then I finally found the strength to let her know it was ok to go. I would be ok. (For the record, I was lying. I had no clue if I would be ok, NONE, but I knew it was likely what she needed to hear). I asked her if she heard me to squeeze my hand, and she squeezed it. I hugged her. I told her I loved her and that I would see her soon, then walked out her room, hugged my dad between tears, and headed to the airport. I prayed the whole flight and for a person who is an avid plane sleeper, I couldn't sleep a wink. Plane landed, turned on my phone and Instagram. My cousin had posted a picture of my grandmother that said, "We will miss you." RAGE entered my veins, and then sadness consumed me. My dad and husband arranged for one of my closest cousins, Marvin, to meet me at the hotel, as their plan was to tell me once I had company. Well that was ruined, but he met me anyway. On one hand, I thought it was so insensitive to post a picture before the whole family was informed, but on the other hand, it didn't change ONE DAMN thing. My grandma had soared to higher heights and was now reunited with my grandpa. It sounded nice, but now I was faced with the reality of doing life without her. What would Sunday dinners become? Who would I talk to every day on the ride home from work for an hour? Who would play "what if" with me for hours and never complain? Who would be my Annapolis Mall shopping buddy? Who would hold all my secrets? Who would tell me when I was wrong but provide unconditional support until I got right? WHO?

October came and my body was WORN OUT and giving out, mentally, physically, emotionally, spiritually. I was sick and didn't even know it. After all, who has time to be sick when you are planning a funeral, working around the clock, active in multiple organizations, and the list goes on. As a Black woman, we are raised to be Superwoman, right? Well, yes, until my primary care physician handed me orders to be off work for 10 weeks. Ten weeks? This must be a joke. I was just promoted. I can't do this. Why do I have to take time off? I'll get more sleep, I'll work remotely three days a week. The negotiations kept going, but he heard none of it. My levels were out of control, and that was the final call. Home. Bed rest. Exercise. Sleep. I'm in my 30s, this can't be life. What will happen to my team, my role, my client groups? (The answer I learned later is NOTHING. Nothing will happen to them. While you are valuable to an organization, business can, will and should continue in your temporary absence. Our health is our responsibility but we often put it to the side to meet the expectations of our role not realizing the long-term implications of our decision and the impact it has on our families. The harsh reality is a company will be ok, but will you?)

Not that I had much choice, I listened to my doctor. I informed my job and followed the orders. A few weeks in, my levels started to regulate. Was it stress? Couldn't be. Again, I'm superwoman, right? Soon I started to realize my grandma was gone in a physical sense but still with me, and she told me to never give up. She told me don't let the office use you because you'll look up one day and realize you gave all you had and got little in return. We opted to try a new doctor that my colleague had told me about for years. He recommended that we take the endometrial receptivity array (ERA) to determine how many days of progesterone we needed before transfer. We got the results back in November and started all the paperwork to transfer our last embryos. Unfortunately, we learned that we would have to transfer with our original doctor because the facility of the new doctor would not accept the embryos the way they were stored/frozen. This was disappointing, but our new doctor assured us he would work with the team on the protocol, and he did just that. We transferred in December and got an early Christmas present on December 23. We were pregnant!!

PREGNANT AGAIN — ROUND 2

Pregnant on vacation looks different: No wine, no whiskey, no hookah, no massages. Nonetheless, we set out to enjoy the sunny beaches of Panama City, Panama. The cherry on top was that my line sister, Katreice and her husband, were scheduled to meet us on our second day. We talked leading up to it and although she had been in and out of the hospital, she was still hopeful that she could make the trip. We arrived, and I confirmed that their hotel room would be right next to ours. The next day she called me to tell me they moved her to hospice, and she just got out. HOSPICE? "Katreice, are you drinking? This is not a good joke." [As background, Katreice had been battling breast cancer and the journey wasn't easy–infection in the port, last- minute cancellation of an important surgery, illness, blood clots. While the list was endless, so was her faith, so we felt confident that it would be a matter of time before we were celebrating remission].

Needless to say, they didn't make the trip. On January 6, I was scheduled to return to work and went for my check-up appointment on the way in for the sonogram. The results: A sac, no baby. Once I stopped the meds, I would miscarry. I was beside myself with grief. I remember the doctor telling me there was still hope, but I was out of embryos and my body didn't respond the last time I tried to collect more. The doctor told me it was ok to take a break, and I could try again or try donor eggs. I remember calling my boss to share the news, but I really don't remember what she said. I called my dad–no heart to call my mom. To be honest, I don't even know if I told her we were pregnant. Who wants to break her heart twice? I left the doctor's office and drove straight to the cemetery to sit with my grandparents. It was 42 degrees, and I didn't even put on my coat. I was numb. I sat there broken and wanting to climb in the grave with them. How could I possibly go through this twice? How could God take my grandmother and my baby? This felt like a cruel and unusual punishment. What in the world did I do to deserve this? The answer is NOTHING, but I didn't feel that way at the time. This was just my journey. Just like we don't deserve all the blessings we receive. The trials are not payback for bad behavior, they just are just part of our story.

I honestly don't remember much of that day or the weeks that followed. I recall my dad being at my house after I left the cemetery. He canceled his work day just to be there. I fell in his arms and cried. I recall opting for a D&C to avoid that traumatic experience of miscarriage , and I know I took another two weeks off of work. I learned. If you recall, I hopped on a flight for work after my first miscarriage. CRAZY. This time, I took time to mourn the loss(es).

I remember talking to Katreice and trying to hide that I was crying. She asked what was wrong and how the process was going, I told her "I'm just tired." She told me to keep going, but she wasn't buying the tears. "So that's it DeShaun?" "Yes, Treice, that's it. Let's talk about you girl, because you're not missing another trip, so let's get it together." Throughout the month, we talked and texted like we usually do. With each check-in, her levels were getting better and they were weaning her off of the oxygen. Once she reached a certain level, she would be able to go home. By the end of January, things were looking good. She should be home by the first week in February!

THREE DEATHS AND NO BABY

February 15, my husband and I got to bear witness to the union of two amazing friends in Cancun. February 16, I woke up to find out Katreice had passed away. I wasn't numb. I literally felt my spirit leave my body. I called Bryce, her husband, and I tried not to cry. My husband, Fernando, tried to hold me, but I just felt sick and touch was going to make me lose it. As usual, into action I went. I had to tell my line, my dean of pledges, my assistant dean of pledges, our college friends–but how? I found my baby brother Donnie at breakfast and just asked him to pray. He prays like nobody's business. Then one of my close line sisters called, and so it began. I don't remember what I said, I just remember hearing what sounded like shock, hurt, and anger all in one. The challenging thing here is Katreice fought this battle in silencefor the most part. With 15 of us on the line, three of us knew. Heavy burden to carry, but there isn't a thing I wouldn't do for my Katreicey-poo. Plus, we have to respect the choices of our loved ones, even if we think differently. Katreice was naturally a private person but in this instance, she just didn't want anyone to look at her with pity . When someone asked about her, I just encouraged them to call her. I pray that they did. It was the random calls that would make her happy. Every now and then, I'd get "DeShaunie-poo, guess who called me…Well shit, you already know, you were probably behind it." We giggled. I changed the subject.

Broken and confused. In the matter of five months, I lost my grandma, my baby, and one of my best friends–my bridesmaid who was supposed to be the godmother to my children. At work, I was *confidentially* informed that it was frowned upon that I took time off following my miscarriage. The irony here was that my miscarriage in itself was *confidential*, so color me crazy when I was floored that my taking time off was even a topic of conversation. I'll spare you the rest of the work disappointment but needless to say, I thought I needed to start 2020 over again. Any reason to hold a small gathering is a good reason! [Note, as a HR executive, I've questioned for years why miscarriages are not consistently covered in most standard bereavement policies. In the US, there are approximately 900,000 to 1 million miscarriages per year. A miscarriage is a death. Perhaps this is something to advocate for in your companies in the future.]

On February 29th (this year was a leap year), we declared it the new New Year's Eve because we needed a re-do on the year. Fernando and I chose to host a small group of friends who are really family. And, my dad and his wife joined us to celebrate his retirement. Sparklers, champagne, food, and laughter–the perfect celebration. Fourteen days later, COVID-19 brought the U.S. to a standstill. Jokes was on us, but it's not a funny one.

SILVER TINT IN THE CLOUDS OF DOUBT

The lives lost during this pandemic were unfortunate and unnecessary. The lives lost at the hands and legs of law enforcement–heartbreaking and unexplainable. I prayed and prayed for these families. Simultaneously, the world slowed down. I slowed down. I found "the silver tint in the clouds of doubt." My peace started to return. I accepted my grandmother being gone; I accepted my baby not getting the chance to exit the womb; I leaned in and held on tighter to Katreice's children, Chris and Joi, while still working on accepting her physical absence. The daily hustle and bustle was gone. I am more productive working from home, so that wasn't a difficult transition. I appreciated not having to sit in traffic for 2.5 hours of each workday. I worked out. I reconnected with my faith. My body returned to normal, as did my inner soul. I began feeling like me again.

August 2021 came and I felt like me again. I felt like I could try again. We started the process. When I got the protocol, I looked at the dates and felt good. My monitoring appointment fell the day before my cousin Nicole's birthday. Transfer would be the day after my mom's birthday, and the results of the transfer would be given on my grandmother's birthday. In my mind, three stars aligned for the three loves that I lost. This would ultimately yield God's most precious gift in human form.

BLESSED YET ANXIOUS

"Do not be anxious about anything, but in
every situation, by prayer and petition with
thanksgiving, present your requests to God."
—Philippians 4:6 NIV

If ever there was a virtue I was missing, it would have been
patience. On this journey, I learned that things would not
happen on my time but rather on God's time. And it did…
finally. The Good Book tells us not to be anxious, however,
here I was 18 weeks pregnant with my son, blessed yet anxious. From rational to completely irrational, I had worries
that ranged the gamut. I worried about whether my relent-
less sneezing would affect the baby. I had a tinge of fear that
I would see blood when I used the restroom. I scaled back
my already inconsistent Peloton workouts for fear of doing
too much. I worried about eating the right things, not eating
enough, or eating too much. I worried about my water intake

and what could happen if I accidentally rolled to my stomach when I was asleep. I worried about how the air pressure in the airplane cabin might affect me. I worried about stressing too much at work and causing another miscarriage. The list goes on.

It is completely possible, and dear I say, human, to be blessed yet anxious. And that was me for some portion of every day. The worrying doesn't stop just because you get pregnant. One could effectively argue that it increases. I didn't have much success in eradicating the worry, but I did learn to shift the energy to prayer when I caught myself.

REBUILDING YOUR SOUL

It is impossible to give your best when you're not at your best. It has taken me quite some time to get this and frankly, I am still learning to apply it consistently. Self-love is not a luxury, it is a responsibility to yourself and those around you. As one who naturally yields to the desires of others, this has been difficult to put into practice. On this journey, it is not a choice, it's a responsibility. I am learning that it is ok to say NO. I am learning that NO is a complete answer —excuse or explanation is not necessary. I am learning that just because you can doesn't mean you should. I am learning that I can't "burn the candles at both ends," as my dad would say, or "You can soar with the eagles at dawn and hoot with the owls at night." I am learning that my energy actually runs out. I am learning that you have to establish boundaries on your time, both at home and at work. I am learning that just because the phone is ringing, it doesn't mean I have to answer it. I am learning that a text message is not an SOS. If it's urgent, they will call...and call again and again. I am learning that it is ok to take a "mental health" day or check into a fancy spa. I am learning it's ok to have a binge day, even if your husband thinks it's crazy. I am learning to do what makes ME happy and what fills my soul. Yes, I still strive to be a loving wife, daughter, daughter-in-law, granddaughter, sister, aunt, godmother, niece, cousin, boss, colleague, sorority sister, and friend. But unless I learn to take care of myself, I will be deflating my value to them and decreasing my time with them.

I've learned so much through this process about myself, my husband, our marriage, and our faith. God uses interesting measures to teach us things but just know, God always keeps his promises. Always.

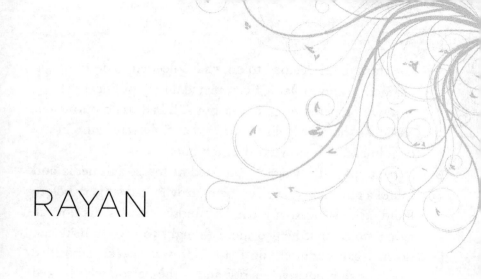

RAYAN

"Our soul waits for the Lord.
He is our help and our shield."
—Psalm 33:20 NIV

I n 2016, we were pregnant with twins. The first one passed at six weeks and the second one at 13 weeks. From that I found out that I had a non-cancerous tumor (acoustic neuroma), and had to have brain surgery to remove it. This took up a lot of my year for recovery. I had to learn to re-swallow and re-balance, go through speech and physical therapy. It was a lot. The first couple of days, I was discouraged because it was so overwhelming trying to learn so much over again. I remember the first day, I didn't want to do it. I was feeling pity for myself and was frustrated. I told the nurse to get out of my room, I wasn't doing anything. I was ready to go home at that point but couldn't go until I was able to master some of the goals they had for me in physical therapy. The next day while sitting in bed, I knew if I didn't do some of these things they were asking, I would not get to go home.

The third day, I decided to do what I needed to do to be discharged. A month later, I completed all my physical therapy and was prepared to go home, but still had to do outpatient sessions. The best feeling during that time was being in my own house, in my own bed. It felt good.

One day after therapy, I looked at my social media and found a guy named Jon Templeman, who had surgery before I did. He changed my whole mindset. It was his encouraging words that helped me. I thought to myself, if he can do it, I can definitely do it too. He was speaking positive words, giving positive energy, and is the person who kicked my butt into gear and believes this too shall pass. Jon's post read something like this: "Your strength is what you make it, and don't let something like this hold you back." Everyday he worked on gaining strength and stability again. This was a positive look on my life.

That same day, I decided I was going to crush my goals at physical therapy and graduate. After half a month, I reached my completion goal. The therapist told me there was really nothing else we could do besides give myself time to heal. I received my graduation certificate, and it was a great feeling. I was on my way to my new norm. By that time, I could drive again due to my blurry vision becoming normal. After 2 and 1/2 months post-op, I started going back to my CrossFit class. It helped with my stability and strength tremendously. I was weak on my left side, so I had to build my strength again. Fitness became my therapeutic moment, and this is why my brand was created–MARKS ON FITNESS.

I started working out years ago with a trainer in Dallas, but later I moved to Jacksonville and found a CrossFit gym. Prior to my surgery, I took fitness for granted once it helped me get to a healthy state and capable of doing things I couldn't do. In 2017, I returned to Texas and started back working out with my old trainer. I realized I had lost a lot of strength over time, so I was determined to get back on track. I was working out but wasn't losing as much weight as I wanted to. I felt uncomfortable and at my heaviest weight, not to mention my health was at stake. In January of 2018, I decided to start a healthy lifestyle journey. I gradually started taking steps to stop drinking sodas and juice to drink more water and eat more vegetables. I started with baby steps so I could lose weight. I went from 175 lbs., which is big for my body frame, to 145 lbs. in a little over a year. I felt like the weight was hindering my health, which was a good reason to lose. Doctors would always say that whenever deciding to have kids, living a healthy lifestyle also helps.

Since the fitness movement, I've been able to gain friendships with a lot of different fitness gurus and trainers. We share our stories on the journey. I also have a private group on Facebook, and a lot of my Texas friends are in that group. Back home, we didn't grow up in a healthy state. We ate what we wanted, and that is all we knew. With the Facebook page, a lot of my classmates and old friends from back home started following and working out themselves. Now I have a couple of people who will post their fitness journey, and there are others who have a private fitness journey but are doing work in the shadows. Every time I start feeling like I should stop posting on my page, someone always sends me a message and tells me how I have inspired them. This gives me motivation to continue. This helps my accountability. Inspiring others on their journey is my encouragement to post on social media.

I am creating a fitness brand legacy and motivating others to live a healthy lifestyle because I grew up not knowing. We only knew the diet that our parents and our grandparents would prepare for us. I want people to know that you can start changing your legacy by eating healthy and making better choices. Not necessarily cutting out everything that you enjoy eating, but making better choices versus what we grew up eating. Life can hit you hard, but that doesn't mean you have to give up. You can take that licking and keep on ticking. God gives his toughest battles to His strongest soldiers.

God won't put anything on you that you cannot bear, and I'm a living witness. To have my husband as a support system means the world to me because he was (and still is) the stronger person in our relationship. He helps me keep moving during my toughest battles, keeps his emotional side to a minimum to spare my feelings, and speaks with positivity. If I could wave a magic wand, I would wish for a healthy pregnancy with no complications, a healthy baby/babies, and a healthy mother.

An Open
Letter to My
Unborn Child

"Before I formed you in the
womb I knew you;
Before you were born
I sanctified you…"
—Jeremiah 1:5 NKJV

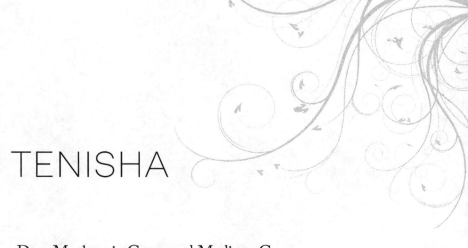

TENISHA

Dear Mackenzie Grace and Madison Grace,

Thank you for making your mama strong, resilient, and patient. I prayed for patience. I prayed for God to make me a better person, and God gave me you. There is not a day or night that I do not think of you. You both are my heartbeats, and I know that you are in heaven with your grandmothers watching over your dad and me. Thank you for loving me more than I could ever love myself. Thank you for forcing me to allow God to use me, and thank you for giving me a stronger purpose.

As I held you in my arms, I knew your spirit would always be with me. I know in my heart you are helping God prepare your siblings for me. I'm sorry that my body failed you. I tried so hard to hold on to you, but God told me to let you go. Please know that I love you, and one day we will meet again.

My loves you are everything, and I know if you're anything like your mama, you are turning up in heaven. Thank you for leading your sister, Banx, to me! I am forever grateful.

I love you both! Forever loves!
Your mom!

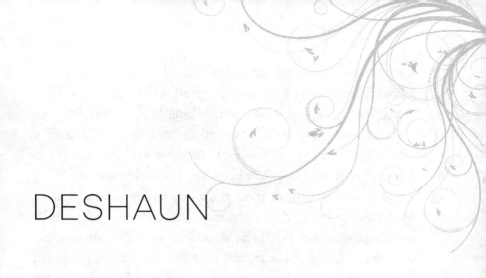

DESHAUN

To my Precious Baby, –

You are my greatest accomplishment and most meaningful blessing. I am so thankful that you are making me a mommy. Mother is a title that only God can give and that no one can take away. Years ago when I thought of being a mommy, a space in my heart was created just for you! I have prayed for this day for so long, and I can't wait for you to make your grand entrance into this world. Your daddy and I already love you beyond measure and look forward to relishing in the mere presence of your being.

Getting to this point has been a JOURNEY, but knowing the joy you will bring to our family and the endless possibilities of your future makes it all worth it. They say "Good things come to those who wait" and you, my sweet child, are worth waiting for. The minute I hold you, I have no doubt that the emptiness of loss, the scars of disappointment, and the moments of sheer hopelessness will all fade away, but the lessons will not. God has truly used the yearning for you to mold, test, and strengthen me and your daddy to ensure you have the parents you need and deserve. In this journey to you, I have learned so much about myself, for which I look forward to sharing with you and instilling those values in you.

In waiting for your conception and successful arrival, firstly, I've learned the value of true love and its role in creating you. Your daddy has been so supportive and uplifting. There is no us without him, and our journey has created an unshakeable bond that only magnifies our story. Secondly, be compassionate to others, as you never know what someone else is going through, but also have grace with yourself. I've learned that taking care of self is equally if not more important. Sleeping, eating, laughing, and meditating are all important to take care of the temple (our body) that God has given us, for it is this body that houses you, our future king or queen of our family. And third, yet most important, is the value of patience and trust in the Lord despite any and all circumstances. He will never fail you or forsake you, and you are a reflection of the love that God has for me and your daddy. Thank you for choosing us to be your parents. While we can't wait to meet you, we will happily and faithfully wait for you!

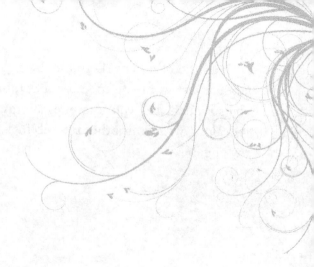

RAYAN

Dear Unborn Child,

You are one of God's greatest gifts to us in this lifetime. I cannot wait to hold, kiss, smell, and touch you. I've waited years to become your mom. God proves his faith every day, even when I'm blind to his word. One day, I will be able to tell you the story of all the struggles and heartaches to have the perfect child that you are. And I cannot wait to tell you about your big sisters, Jade (my bonus big girl) and Rylee (my amazing angel baby). Mommy and daddy will love you always.

BONUS LETTER: TO MY BORN CHILD

To my dearest Rylee,

I miss you like crazy!!! Not a day goes by that I don't think of kissing and holding you in my arms. Some days are harder than other days without you. I hope you are playing with all the other angels and looking down on us with a big smile. I just want you to know that mommy and daddy love you so much. Tell your grannies and grandpas we love them too, along with your other two siblings there with you. R.I.P. my angel.

CONCLUSION

I f you remember nothing else that you have read amidst the pages of this book, know that you are not alone. There are others living this life as well. This doesn't just happen to women on their own, but it is happening throughout the world, as there are millions of women who are having this issue. With every passing day, more and more women are coming forth. It is important for us to speak up about this because so many suffer in silence. When we resolve to speak more, we can find peace. It is therapeutic. Being transparent about our stories, our friendship, and most importantly our faith, has changed each of us for the better. And for this reason, we have resolved to share the gift of Faith, Friendship, and Fertility with you.

ABOUT THE AUTHORS

Tenisha Patterson Brown, Esq., is a business and legal consultant for athletes and entrepreneurs, entrepreneur, philanthropist, wife, and mother. As a serial entrepreneur and consultant, Tenisha has spent most of her adult life learning and working to build her clients' brands and her brand. Shortly after getting married, she embarked on a journey of vulnerability, bringing awareness to the struggles of infertility and pregnancy loss. Her brand not only captures the importance of reproductive health but also building strong marriages, as evidenced in the books she co-authored, *100 Ways to Stay Married*, and *the Success and Submission Community*. Her greatest passion is to speak life into others and her daughter Banx.

DeShaun N. Wise Porter is a human resources executive for a Fortune 500 Company, a wife, a mother, and a philanthropist. As the global head of diversity, equity, inclusion and engagement, DeShaun's work centers on building a diverse workforce through transformational talent initiatives and equitable programs. Outside of her corporate setting,

DeShaun is a world traveler with a passion for helping to educate, develop, and empower others to be their authentic selves through her work with youth. Albeit a private person, she quickly learned that her testimony with infertility could help others overcome the obstacles by embracing *faith over fear.*

Rayan Marks is a fitness influencer, lifestyle blogger, and entrepreneur. A graduate of DeVry University's Computer Technology Department, Rayan is on a mission to impact the world through the intersection of fitness, food, health, and community-driven accountability, inspiring women to achieve their highest potential. A serial entrepreneur, brand owner, and mom, Rayan knows firsthand the health struggles women face as a pre-eclampsia and acoustic neuroma survivor. Her brand Marks On Fitness, created in 2019, seeks to empower women to take control of their health and happiness at any age.

MOMS IN WAITING

Take this space to reflect on your experiences with pregnancy. This is not a space to feel like you have to be perfect. LET IT OUT!

List your support systems. How have they kept you strong?

_____

_____

_____

_____

_____

_____

_____

_____

_____

_____

_____

_____

_____

PATTERSON, WISE, & MARKS

Talk about a time when you wanted to give up on this journey. Why didn't you?

_____

_____

_____

_____

_____

_____

_____

_____

_____

_____

_____

_____

_____

What are some things you like to do for yourself to encourage self-care?

At this chapter in your life, what are you grateful for?

_____

_____

_____

_____

_____

_____

_____

_____

_____

_____

_____

_____

_____

Faith, Friendship, and Fertility Movement

WHO WE ARE

We are a community of survivors and thrivers. We are a family that unites to support, uplift, and guide individuals and families through the journey of becoming parents.

WHAT WE DO

Our goal is to transform the conversation and to provide financial support to individuals and families struggling with infertility.

HOW TO GET INVOLVED

Follow us on social media:

INSTAGRAM
@FAITHFRIENDSHIPFERTILITY

FACEBOOK
@FAITHFRIENDSHIPFERTILITY

WEBSITE:
WWW.FAITHFRIENDSHIPFERTILITY.COM
AND SUBSCRIBE FOR OUR UPDATES

Join us for our annual **Faith, Friendship and Fertility Conference!** Visit our website for dates and location information.

Printed in the USA
CPSIA information can be obtained
at www.ICGtesting.com
JSHW011706050923
47829JS00010B/28

9 781953 156402